AMERICAN JOURNAL of PUBLIC HEALTH
SEPTEMBER 2023
Issue 9

AJPH

A PUBLICATION OF THE
AMERICAN PUBLIC HEALTH ASSOCIATION

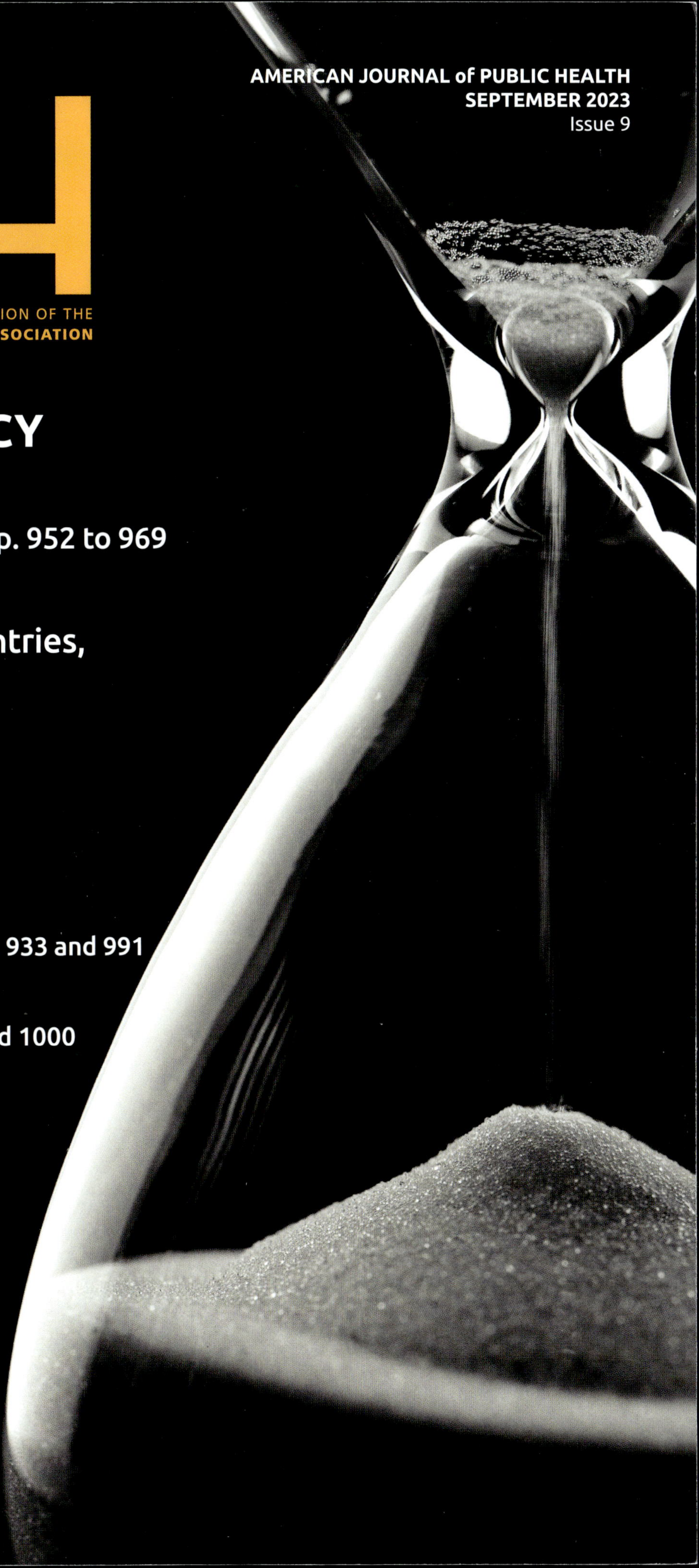

US LIFE EXPECTANCY FALLING BEHIND

Failing Population Health, pp. 952 to 969

Role of Education, p. 964

United States vs Other Countries, 1933–2021, p. 970

Also in this issue:

HISTORY
Children and Pandemics, p. 985

OVERDOSE TRENDS
US State-Level Differences, pp. 933 and 991

PUBLIC HEALTH WORKFORCE
Promoting Diversity, pp. 936 and 1000

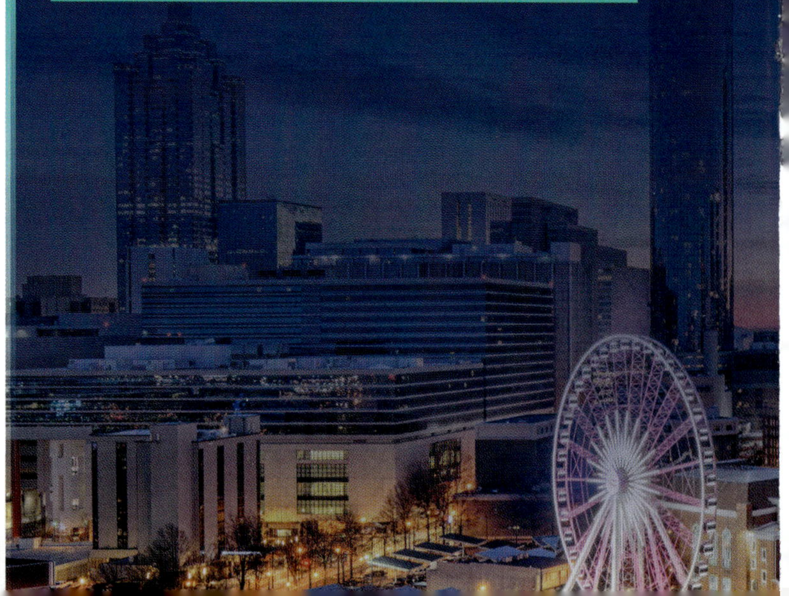

APHA
AMERICAN PUBLIC HEALTH ASSOCIATION
For science. For action. For health.

AJPH®, published monthly, is the official Journal of the American Public Health Association®, 800 I St NW, Washington, DC 20001-3710; (202) 777- APHA; TDD (202) 777-2500. APHA is a nongovernmental professional society founded in 1872, representing all disciplines and specialties in public health.

The *American Journal of Public Health*® (*AJPH*) (print ISSN: 0090-0036; electronic ISSN: 1541- 0048), first published in 1911, is the official journal of the American Public Health Association® (APHA). The oldest and largest organization of public health professionals in the world, APHA represents approximately 30 000 members from more than 50 occupations of public health.

Submissions: Visit www.editorialmanager.com/ajph or ajph.edmgr.com for online manuscript preparation and submission guidelines. Contributions of original unpublished research, social science analyses, scholarly essays, critical commentaries, departments, and letters to the editor are welcome. Questions? Write ajph.submissions@apha.org or call APHA at (202) 777-2469.

Print plus online subscriptions: Institutional price (print copy with online access for a single institution and all authorized users, regardless of geographic location) varies by size of organization and ranges from $993–$1445 for US organizations, and $1073–$1526 for international organizations (air delivery); multiple campuses not permitted without special arrangement. Details of the tiered pricing system at https://subscriptionoffice.com/pages/apha-landing-page. To order, write apha.subscriptions@apha.org.

Online-only subscriptions: Institutional price for one institution and its authorized users (regardless of geographic location) is $878–$1307. To order, write apha.subscriptions@apha.org. For academic consortia or multisite corporate subscriptions, contact apha.subscriptions@apha.org.

Print-only subscriptions: Institutional price is US $701, $782 international.

Back print issues: A limited number of print issues are for sale. Single copies are US $49, $55 international (air delivery). Shipping included; prepay only. To order, write apha.subscriptions@apha.org.

Reprints: For prices and ordering information on 50 or more reprints, check the Reprints section at www.ajph.org. To order smaller quantities of reprints (rush delivery), use the "Purchase Article" link on the article site itself.

Electronic access: Online articles more than 10 years old are available free for personal use at www.ajph.org. Recent articles are available through pay-per-view: single PDF article for $24, single issue access for 24 hours for $33, or entire site access for 24 hours for $38.

Postal information: Periodicals postage paid at Washington, DC, and additional mailing offices. Postmaster: Send address changes to American Journal of Public Health, 800 I St NW, Washington, DC 20001-3710.

Address changes: Send to AJPH, Membership Department (members) or AJPH Subscriptions (subscribers), APHA, 800 I St NW, Washington, DC 20001-3710. Or write to membership.mail@apha. org (members) or apha.subscriptions@apha.org (subscribers).

Advertising: For pricing and other information, see www.ajph.org. Please write to ashell.alston@apha.org or call (202) 777-2470 for other advertising opportunities. Ask about special exhibit packages and sponsorships. Acceptance of advertising by the *Journal* does not imply endorsement of products.

Indexes: Publications that index or abstract articles from AJPH include the following: Ageline, Assia (Applied Social Science Index and Abstracts), Biological Abstracts, Chemical Abstracts, CINAHL, Criminal Justice Abstracts, EMBASE, EMCare, Environmental Abstracts, e-psyche, ERIC, ETOH (Alcohol and Alcohol Problems Science Database), Excerpta Medica, Food Science and Technology, General Science Index, Grateful Med, Hospital Literature Index, Human Resources Abstracts, International Pharmaceutical Abstracts (IPA), Medline, Physical Education Index, Pollution Abstracts, Psychological Abstracts, PsychINFO, Safety Science Abstracts, Sage Family Studies Abstracts, Sage Human Resources Abstracts, Science Citation Index, SCOPUS, SIIC Data Bases, Social Work Research and Abstracts, and Statistical Reference Index (SRI)/LexisNexis.

AJPH

A PUBLICATION OF THE
AMERICAN PUBLIC HEALTH ASSOCIATION

COVER: Life expectancy in the United States has steadily worsened since the 1950s. Globally diverse countries continue to outperform the United States. In this issue of *AJPH*, we explore how US policies and geographic factors may be contributing to this trend.

Cover concept and selection by Aleisha Kropf. Photo by artistseer/iStock. Printed with permission.

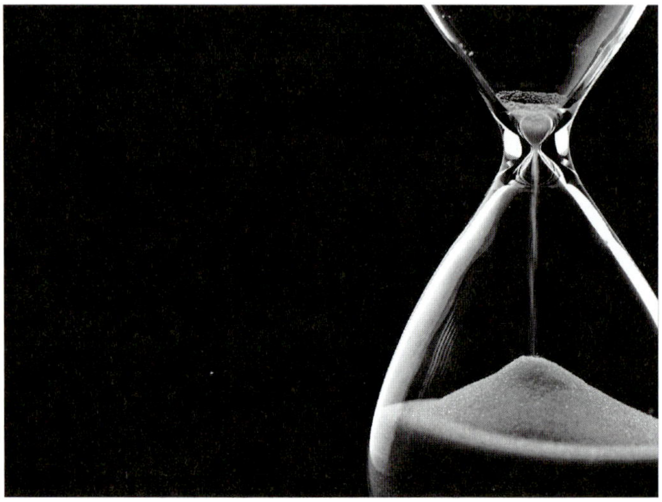

APHA
AMERICAN PUBLIC HEALTH ASSOCIATION
For science. For action. For health.

Promoting public health research, policy, practice, and education is the *AJPH* mission. As we widen our scope to embrace global issues, we also sharpen our focus to support the needs of public health practitioners. We invite contributions of original unpublished research, opinion and commentary, and letters to the editor.

The *Journal* is printed on acid-free recycled paper.

OPEN ACCESS ONLINE ONLY PODCAST DATA SUPPLEMENT AVAILABLE

EDITOR'S CHOICE

932 South Pole 2020: The Year Without COVID-19
H. Rodenberg

OPINIONS, IDEAS, & PRACTICE

EDITORIALS

933 Overdoses, Reproductive Justice, and Harm Reduction
H. L. F. Cooper, W. Rice, J. Cummings, M. D. Livingston, S. Peddireddy, E. Rogers, A. Dunlop, M. Kramer, and N. D. Hernandez

936 Health Equity Requires Public Health Workforce Diversity and Inclusivity: A Public Health of Consequence, September 2023
F. Kapadia

NOTES FROM THE FIELD

939 Hospital-Based Community Gardens as a Strategic Partner in Addressing Community Health Needs
D. R. George and A. E. Ethridge

943 A Mortality Surveillance Collaboration Between a Health System and Public Health Department
S. A. Simpson, R. Loh, L. Elliott, R. Everhart, C. Bass, K. Bol, S. Boylls, and L. Podewils

947 Timely Second-Dose Completion of mRNA COVID-19 Vaccination at Community-Based and Mobile Vaccine Clinics in Maryland
C. Parent, B. F. Bigelow, S. D. Sisson, D. Martínez, C. Yang, and K. R. Page

US LIFE EXPECTANCY

952 An Alarming Trend in US Population Health
K. Rochel de Camargo

954 Trends in Life Expectancy: Learning From International Comparisons
M. P. Farina

956 Trends in US Life Expectancy: Falling Behind and Failing to Act
P. L. Remington

959 Failing Population Health: US Life Expectancy Falling Behind
L. Gaydosh

961 A Deadly Drop in Rankings: How the United States Was Left Behind in Global Life Expectancy Trends
L. Shanahan and W. E. Copeland

964 Something Related to Education May Hold the Key to Understanding What Is Ailing the United States
A. Case

967 The Gap Between US and Best Practice Life Expectancy Is Increasing
J. M. Aburto and S. Vigezzi

RESEARCH & ANALYSIS

US LIFE EXPECTANCY

970 Falling Behind: The Growing Gap in Life Expectancy Between the United States and Other Countries, 1933–2021
S. H. Woolf

CLIMATE CHANGE

981 Ambient Temperature and Emergency Hospital Admissions in People Experiencing Homelessness: London, United Kingdom, 2011–2019
S. Hajat, C. E. Sarran, M. Bezgrebelna, and S. A. Kidd

HISTORY

985 Lessons Ignored: Children and Pandemics
C. Connolly and J. Golden

SURVEILLANCE

991 State-Level History of Overdose Deaths Involving Stimulants in the United States, 1999–2020
D. Kline, A. M. Bunting, S. A. Hepler, A. Rivera-Aguirre, N. Krawczyk, and M. Cerda

1000 Diversity of the US Public Health Workforce Pipeline (2016–2020): Role of Academic Institutions
A. Vichare, Y. H. Park, and C. M. Plepys

OPEN-THEMED RESEARCH

1009 Self-Reported Barriers to Care Among Sexual and Gender Minority People With Disabilities: Findings From The PRIDE Study, 2019–2020
S. Lamba, J. Obedin-Maliver, J. Mayo, A. Flentje, M. E. Lubensky, Z. Dastur, and M. R. Lunn

1019 Benefits of Frequent HIV Testing in the THRIVE Demonstration Project: United States, 2015–2020
A. A. Kimball, W. Zhu, L. Yu, M. R. Tanner, K. Iqbal, K. L. Dominguez, A. Shankar, K. Drezner, K. Musgrove, E. Mayes, W. T. Robinson, C. Schumacher, K. P. Delaney, K. W. Hoover, and the THRIVE Project Team

BACKMATTER

ERRATA

1028 Erratum In: "Beyond #StopAAPIHate: Expanding the Definition of Violence Against Asian Americans"

OTHER DEPARTMENTS

1032 Subscription Form

South Pole 2020: The Year Without COVID-19

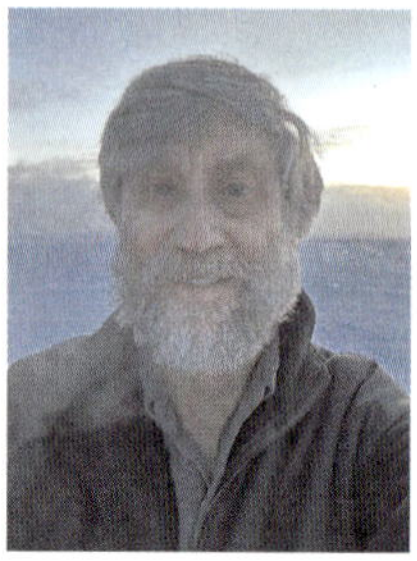

Many of us vividly recall the first year of the COVID-19 pandemic. I was fortunate to work apart from the worst of it, and my family was spared, so my memories are not so much of fear but a house full of kids, LEGO train sets, hassle-free airports, and a weekend road trip to score toilet paper. But there was never any doubt that COVID-19 lay right outside the door, waiting to pounce on those who dropped their guard.

For one group of people, the first year of COVID-19 simply didn't happen. I'm currently spending the austral winter as the physician at the National Science Foundation Amundsen-Scott South Pole Station, and several of my colleagues were here during those critical days of 2020. For them, COVID was simply something they heard about; as a friend said, "It was like reading *The Walking Dead*." They knew about it, got some smidgeons of information, but couldn't see, feel, or experience the crisis in real-time media or in their lives.

"Polies" first heard about COVID in late February, after the station had already closed for the season. (Although a small crew lives at the station during the winter months, the station is physically inaccessible from the outside world from mid-February to mid-October each year.) From a distance, COVID seemed to be just one of a series of catastrophes that year, including the aftermath of the George Floyd incident, nationwide conflicts between protestors and police, and a bitterly contested election. There were deep concerns about the health of family and friends and anxiety from the inability to help or simply be present in a time of need. "We didn't know what we were coming back to," said another workmate. "Was everything going to be burned down when we got back?" With limited information, it was easy to predict the worst.

But as the over-winter staff was effectively isolated before the pandemic was declared, life went on as normal (as normal as it can be when a "good" winter's day is clear and only −60° F). There were no lockdowns, isolation, masking, or social distancing. Indeed, when the 42 stalwart Polies gathered together on March 17, it was likely the largest social event on the planet.

In the latter part of the year, COVID was taken more seriously as preparations were made to transition to the summer crew. Medical staff kept the crew updated as to clinical developments on the outside, and plans were made to accommodate staffing changes. But there was still an element of disbelief if not levity; there were mask-making parties in the arts and crafts room, and the crew "practiced" wearing masks and social distancing for a day.

The full impact of the pandemic was not really felt until those coming to the continent for the following polar summer were subject to prolonged delays from a paucity of flights and isolation in both the United States and New Zealand, confined to hotel rooms except for limited periods of exercise in fenced-off yards. Polies returning to the world, fully educated about strict masking and social distancing, were surprised to find that upon arrival in New Zealand no one else was wearing a mask, as that nation had effectively quarantined itself in the early phases of the pandemic.

COVID-19 finally arrived in Antarctica in 2021 and at the South Pole the following year. The National Science Foundation now has a continental infection control plan in place; my first two weeks on continent were spent in varying degrees of isolation with frequent antigen testing. Antarctica is now in tune with the rest of the world. But at the South Pole, 2020 was not an *annus horribilis*. It was the site of the biggest St. Patrick's Day party in the world. AJPH

Howard Rodenberg, MD, MPH
National Science Foundation/
United States Antarctic Program
Amundsen-Scott South Pole Station, Antarctica

DOI: https://doi.org/10.2105/AJPH.2023.307361

12 Years Ago

Contribution of Obesity to International Differences in Life Expectancy

Life expectancy in the United States has fallen below that of most other industrialized countries and ranked 32nd in the world in 2008. As President Obama has noted, the relatively low level of life expectancy in the United States coexists with the highest per capita expenditure on health care in the world. Explanations of the low US ranking range from a history of high levels of cigarette smoking to low levels of physical activity, a poorly performing health care sector, high levels of income inequality, and high levels of obesity. Identifying the responsible factors would help to clarify the critical public health domains where the United States has fallen furthest behind its peers. . . . We conclude that even when relatively low mortality risks associated with obesity are used, the high levels of obesity in the United States contribute substantially—in the neighborhood of 30%—to the lower level of longevity in the United States. . . . We believe that this demonstration should add urgency to public health efforts aimed at achieving healthier weights for Americans.

From AJPH, November 2011, pp. 2137, 2143.

45 Years Ago

Improving Life Expectancy: An Uphill Road Ahead

If a general cure for cancer were discovered and applied this month, there would be about 30,000 fewer deaths next month, and nearly 350,000 fewer next year. Mortality would seem to be permanently lowered by one-sixth and life expectation increased by one-sixth. . . . [But] if the people who are rescued from cancer are at high risk from heart disease and other causes, then that greatly diminishes the number of years added to human life by the discovery of a cancer cure. . . . Is an expectation of 80 years the intrinsic ceiling against which medicine is pressing? Is future progress to consist solely in extending present achievements to less favored groups? Important as it is to do this, we cannot easily reconcile ourselves to a condition where progress on the frontier suddenly comes to an end. What will be needed, then, to break through the barrier that now seems to be set at about 80 years if "mere" eradication of cancer does not even come close to doing it? The coincidence in age of the presently remaining causes of death suggests that, beyond attacking the individual causes, future research should focus on what underlies them all.

From AJPH, October 1978, pp. 954–956.

Overdoses, Reproductive Justice, and Harm Reduction

Hannah L. F. Cooper, ScD, Whitney Rice, DrPH, Janet Cummings, PhD, Melvin D. Livingston, PhD, Snigdha Peddireddy, MPH, Erin Rogers, MPH, Anne Dunlop, MD, Michael Kramer, PhD, and Natalie D. Hernandez, PhD

ABOUT THE AUTHORS

Hannah L. F. Cooper, Whitney Rice, Melvin D. Livingston, and Snigdha Peddireddy are with the Department of Behavioral, Social, and Health Education Sciences, Rollins School of Public Health, Emory University, Atlanta, GA. Janet Cummings is with the Department of Health Policy and Management, Rollins School of Public Health. Erin Rogers and Michael Kramer are with the Department of Epidemiology, Rollins School of Public Health. Anne Dunlop is with the Department of Obstetrics and Gynecology, School of Medicine, Emory University. Natalie D. Hernandez is with the Center for Maternal Health Equity Community Health and Preventive Medicine, Morehouse School of Medicine, Atlanta, GA.

See also Kline et al., p. 991.

In this issue of *AJPH*, Kline et al. (p. 991) share essential learnings about the fourth wave of the US opioid overdose epidemic that look beyond national and regional patterns to state-specific variations in these deaths. Their landmark analyses reveal significant state-level heterogeneities in suffering during a sweeping 20-year period, including surging rates of fatal psychostimulant and opioid overdoses in West Virginia and Kentucky after 2015 and exceedingly high rates of cocaine-involved deaths in Washington, DC. Each uptick in overdose rates depicted in the authors' Figure 1 represents a staggering loss, as communities mourn family members, friends, and neighbors.

Yet, even these geographically refined data are themselves aggregations across heterogeneous subpopulations. We dedicate this editorial to one population living at a particular intersection of race, ethnicity, sex, and life course: non-Hispanic Black ("Black") pregnant or postpartum people who use drugs (PWUD). These PWUD are fighting to survive at the intersection of two of the gravest 21st-century US public health epidemics: (1) overdoses, and (2) maternal mortality. The United States has the highest maternal mortality rate of all high-income countries, and Black pregnant or postpartum people are approximately three times more likely to die than are their non-Hispanic White ("White") counterparts.[1,2] Overdoses are a leading cause of maternal deaths in multiple states, particularly in the later months of the postpartum year,[3] and the rate of drug-related maternal deaths increased 81% between 2017 and 2020, more than twice the increase in the rate among reproductive-aged women.[4]

Historically, maternal overdose deaths have been concentrated among White people,[5] paralleling patterns in the general population. This historical pattern is, however, shifting, and in recent years overdose mortality rates among Black people in the general population have exceeded those among White people.[6] Overdoses are now the fourth leading cause of death among Black women,[7] and in multiple states maternal overdose death rates among Black pregnant or postpartum people now exceed or equal those among White pregnant or postpartum people.[8,9]

Although US public health agencies and community-based organizations have mobilized to curb epidemics of overdoses and of maternal mortality, these mobilizations have been siloed, and pregnant or postpartum PWUD are falling through the cracks. To illustrate, states have formed maternal mortality review committees that are charged with conducting a social autopsy of each preventable maternal death to identify its cause and make recommendations to ensure that this cause drives no future maternal deaths. As recently as 2019, however, multiple state committees still deemed overdoses "not preventable" and thus outside their scope.[9] Likewise, access to substance use disorder treatment programs offering specialty services for pregnant people remains inadequate (e.g., in 2018, just 23% of substance use disorder treatment programs offered these services).[10]

POSSIBLE POLICY DRIVERS

Kline et al. call for research on the role of state policies in driving overdose deaths. A common public health saying is that each overdose is a policy failure. We raise the possibility instead that each maternal overdose among Black PWUD reveals that our racialized capitalist policies are working as intended. To consider this possibility, we meld harm reduction and reproductive justice approaches. Although historically

AJPH September 2023, Vol 113, No. 9

siloed, these approaches are highly complementary (Box A, available as a supplement to the online version of this article at http://www.ajph.org). Complementarities include centering structural drivers (e.g., policies) that interlock to forge complex social positions and to shape distributions of health and disease across these social positions, honoring and analyzing resistance, and conceptualizing research itself as a form of resistance that members of affected communities must guide. Indeed, a community advisory board of people with histories of using drugs while pregnant or postpartum identified select laws, which we describe in the next sections.

Laws Governing Drug Use in Pregnancy

Although public health research and practice neglect pregnant and postpartum PWUD, state lawmakers set their sights on them: 44 states have enacted at least one law governing drug use in pregnancy (Box B, available as a supplement to the online version of this article at http://www.ajph.org). Many of these laws are openly punitive (e.g., laws requiring that health care providers report pregnant PWUD to child protective services). Part of the war on drugs, these laws have roots in the racialized and gendered "crack baby" panic of the 1980s that framed Black women as unfit mothers willing to sacrifice their children to their all-consuming addiction.[11]

These laws are devastating extensions of reproductive injustices committed during slavery, when slave owners tore families apart by selling Black children as commodities.[12] Then, as now, child removal was inflicted as punishment for "bad" parental behavior. Then, as now, the reach of these reproductive injustices extended far beyond those who actually lost children: the specter of such removals stalked and terrorized Black parents.[12] Consonant with their terrorizing purpose, these putatively race-neutral laws are hyperenforced against Black parents, from obstetricians, who are far more likely to test and report their Black patients for drugs, to child protective service workers, who are far more likely to remove the children of Black parents for drug-related causes.[13]

Research suggests that these removals devastate PWUD: punitive laws governing drug use in pregnancy are associated with a 45% increase in maternal overdoses.[14] Notably, however, research on these ubiquitous policies is still new and rarely focuses specifically on Black pregnant or postpartum people or on resistance strategies they might implement to retain custody or prevent a subsequent overdose.

Abortion Rights

The escalating decimation of abortion rights is similarly intertwined with the war on drugs and may disproportionately increase overdoses among Black postpartum PWUD. Antebellum policies grotesquely conceptualized fetuses—including yet to be conceived fetuses—of enslaved people as property of their White owners that could be willed and inherited separately from the birthing parent.[12] War on drugs era laws governing drug use in pregnancy hew to this legal framework, sacrificing maternal rights—in practice, overwhelmingly Black maternal rights—to fetal personhood. Fetal personhood arguments are, in turn, foundational to antiabortion laws. The resulting escalations in forced birth will fall most heavily on Black people, who have historically exercised their right to abortion more than White people.[12] As *Roe v Wade* falls, essential research is needed on the impact of racialized erosions to abortion rights—and resistance to these erosions—on Black maternal overdoses, given that Black pregnant PWUD will face severe constraints to exercising this right and that these same PWUD will be at high risk for child removal.

Entitlements

Ongoing racialized and gendered erosions of government entitlements may also drive maternal overdoses among impoverished Black PWUD. The safety net woven in the 20th century to prevent malnutrition and houselessness by Temporary Assistance for Needy Families; the Special Supplemental Nutrition Program for Women, Infants, and Children; subsidized housing; the Supplemental Nutrition Assistance Program; and other entitlements was built to support White families and has systematically abandoned Black families.[15,16] The war on drugs worsened this abandonment, when federal and state governments excluded people with felony convictions, and sometimes specifically drug-related felony convictions, from these protections. These exclusions arose only after racialized criminal–legal systems had hyperenforced punitive drug laws against Black individuals. Given that houselessness and malnutrition create physiological and social vulnerability to overdoses,[17,18] a key but currently unexamined question is whether these exclusions—which are elements of a highly effective policy framework supporting White supremacy—generate overdoses among Black pregnant or postpartum women.

Reproductive justice advocates have successfully sought to extend Medicaid through the postpartum year in many states, and Medicaid is a bedrock of overdose prevention because it covers substance use disorder treatment. Unfortunately, people who are incarcerated for more than a month lose their Medicaid coverage, and many struggle to reenroll upon release. Because of racialized criminal–legal systems, Black PWUD are disproportionately more likely to be incarcerated for prolonged periods. Pressing, but as yet unexamined, questions are whether postpartum expansion reduces maternal overdoses and whether its effects are attenuated among Black pregnant or postpartum people.

CONCLUSIONS

The landmark article by Kline et al. opens new vistas for analyses of state-level heterogeneities in, and thus determinants of, the opioid overdose epidemic's fourth wave. Reproductive justice and harm reduction approaches demand that this and related research center pregnant or postpartum Black PWUD, who are struggling to survive at the intersection of the ongoing and dynamic opioid overdose crisis, the US maternal mortality crisis, and racialized capitalism. AJPH

CORRESPONDENCE

Correspondence should be sent to Hannah L. F. Cooper, 1518 Clifton Rd, NE, Atlanta, GA 30322 (e-mail: hcoope3@sph.emory.edu). Reprints can be ordered at http://www.ajph.org by clicking the "Reprints" link.

PUBLICATION INFORMATION

Full Citation: Cooper HLF, Rice W, Cummings J, et al. Overdoses, reproductive justice, and harm reduction. *Am J Public Health*. 2023;113(9): 933–935.

Acceptance Date: June 27, 2023.

DOI: https://doi.org/10.2105/AJPH.2023.307379

CONTRIBUTORS

H. L. F. Cooper conceptualized and drafted the editorial. W. Rice, E. Rogers, A. Dunlop, M. Kramer, and N. D. Hernandez led the application of the reproductive justice framework. J. Cummings, M. D. Livingston, and S. Peddireddy led the application of the harm reduction framework. All authors reviewed and revised the editorial.

ACKNOWLEDGMENTS

We are grateful to our funders, which include the Center for Reproductive Health Research in the Southeast, funded through an anonymous foundation (grants R01DA058065, T32DA050552, R01DA046197I).

CONFLICTS OF INTEREST

The authors have no conflicts of interest to declare.

REFERENCES

1. Joseph KS, Boutin A, Lisonkova S, et al. Maternal mortality in the United States: recent trends, current status, and future considerations. *Obstet Gynecol*. 2021;137(5):763–771. https://doi.org/10.1097/AOG.0000000000004361
2. Centers for Disease Control and Prevention. Racial/ethnic disparities in pregnancy-related deaths—United States, 2007–2016. *MMWR Morb Mortal Wkly Rep*. 2019;68(35):762–765. https://doi.org/10.15585/mmwr.mm6835a3
3. Schiff DM, Nielsen T, Terplan M, et al. Fatal and nonfatal overdose among pregnant and postpartum women in Massachusetts. *Obstet Gynecol*. 2018;132(2):466–474. https://doi.org/10.1097/AOG.0000000000002734
4. Bruzelius E, Martins SS. US trends in drug overdose mortality among pregnant and postpartum persons, 2017–2020. *JAMA*. 2022;328(21):2159–2161. https://doi.org/10.1001/jama.2022.17045
5. Margerison CE, Roberts MH, Gemmill A, Goldman-Mellor S. Pregnancy-associated deaths due to drugs, suicide, and homicide in the United States, 2010–2019. *Obstet Gynecol*. 2022; 139(2):172–180. https://doi.org/10.1097/AOG.0000000000004649
6. Friedman JR, Hansen H. Evaluation of increases in drug overdose mortality rates in the US by race and ethnicity before and during the COVID-19 pandemic. *JAMA Psychiatry*. 2022;79(4):379–381. https://doi.org/10.1001/jamapsychiatry.2022.0004
7. Harris RA, Mandell DS. Years of life lost to drug overdose among Black female individuals in the US, 2015–2021. *JAMA Psychiatry*. 2023;80(3): 276–277. https://doi.org/10.1001/jamapsychiatry.2022.4194
8. Goldman-Mellor S, Margerison CE. Maternal drug-related death and suicide are leading causes of postpartum death in California. *Am J Obstet Gynecol*. 2019;221(5):489.e1–489.e9. https://doi.org/10.1016/j.ajog.2019.05.045
9. Smid MC, Stone N, Baksh L, et al. Pregnancy-associated death in Utah: contribution of drug-induced deaths. *Obstet Gynecol*. 2019;133(6):1131–1140. https://doi.org/10.1097/AOG.0000000000003279
10. Meinhofer A, Hinde JM, Ali MM. Substance use disorder treatment services for pregnant and postpartum women in residential and outpatient settings. *J Subst Abuse Treat*. 2020;110:9–17. https://doi.org/10.1016/j.jsat.2019.12.005
11. Zerai A, Banks R. *Dehumanizing Discourse, Anti-Drug Law, and Policy in America: A "Crack Mother's" Nightmare*. New York, NY: Ashgate Press; 2002.
12. Roberts DE. *Killing the Black Body: Race, Reproduction, and the Meaning of Liberty*. New York, NY: Vintage Books; 2017.
13. Cénat JM, McIntee S-E, Mukunzi JN, Noorishad P-G. Overrepresentation of Black children in the child welfare system: a systematic review to understand and better act. *Child Youth Serv Rev*. 2021;120:105714. https://doi.org/10.1016/j.childyouth.2020.105714
14. Tabatabaeepour N, Morgan JR, Jalali A, Kapadia SN, Meinhofer A. Impact of prenatal substance use policies on commercially insured pregnant females with opioid use disorder. *J Subst Abuse Treat*. 2022;140:108800. https://doi.org/10.1016/j.jsat.2022.108800
15. Gordon L. *Pitied but Not Entitled: Single Mothers and the History of Welfare, 1890–1935*. New York, NY: Free Press; 1994.
16. Quadagno J. *The Color of Welfare: How Racism Undermined the War on Poverty*. New York, NY: Oxford University Press; 1994.
17. Pérez-Figueroa RE, Obonyo DJ, Santoscoy S, et al. Housing instability, structural vulnerability, and non-fatal opioid overdoses among people who use heroin in Washington Heights, New York City. *Behav Med*. 2022;48(4):320–330. https://doi.org/10.1080/08964289.2021.1922347
18. Yamamoto A, Needleman J, Gelberg L, Kominski G, Shoptaw S, Tsugawa Y. Association between homelessness and opioid overdose and opioid-related hospital admissions/emergency department visits. *Soc Sci Med*. 2019;242:112585. https://doi.org/10.1016/j.socscimed.2019.112585

Health Equity Requires Public Health Workforce Diversity and Inclusivity: A Public Health of Consequence, September 2023

Farzana Kapadia, PhD, MPH

ABOUT THE AUTHOR

Farzana Kapadia is the deputy editor of AJPH *and is a professor of epidemiology at the School of Global Public Health, New York University, New York.*

See also Vichare et al., p. 1000.

AJPH September 2023, Vol 113, No. 9

In the October 1923 issue of *AJPH*, Winslow et al. published a report enumerating the handful of public health degrees conferred by the 10 US institutions providing education in public health.[1] Although we have no data on the student population receiving these degrees, the report does note that they were most often awarded to those who had already attained either an undergraduate or medical degree between 1921 and 1922—a predominantly White and male population. Fast forward to 2023, and there are now hundreds of schools and programs of public health across the United States awarding more than 20 different types of undergraduate and graduate public health degrees (https://programfinder.aspph.org). This growth in public health schools and programs, especially in the past 20 years, is a reflection of several factors. These include the growth of public health employment opportunities across public and private sectors[2] as well as a response to the growing range of acute health crises (e.g., COVID-19, Zika, etc.) as well as chronic public health (e.g., obesity, substance use disorders, HIV, etc.) issues affecting population health. In the US, public health professionals address public health crises rooted in systems of structural racism and socioeconomic inequalities as well as rising tides of xenophobia and lesbian, gay, bisexual, transgender, and queer (LGBTQ+) discrimination: the growing inequalities in life expectancy, persistently high maternal and infant mortality rates, the opioid overdose epidemic, the attacks on reproductive justice, the gun violence pandemic, and the attacks on LGBTQ+ rights, to name just a few. Responsiveness to these myriad yet equally pressing health challenges requires that all public health professionals are trained not only to be deeply and truly cognizant of the needs of the communities they serve but to have a clear and cogent understanding of the social and structural drivers that fuel health inequalities within and across populations. Thus, attention to the pipeline that produces our public health workforce and ensuring that the pipeline is diverse across multiple factors is crucial. Equally important is ensuring that this workforce is appropriately trained to address the multilevel factors that fuel our public health challenges.

MEASURING DIVERSITY IN THE PIPELINE

In this issue of *AJPH*, Vichare et al. (p. 1000) present an interesting approach to quantifying diversity in schools and programs of public health. By comparing the proportion of minority graduates, defined in this study as Black, Hispanic/Latinx, Native Hawaiian and Pacific Islanders, and American Indian and Alaska Natives, at accredited public health schools and programs to the proportion of those same minority persons in the state where that institution is located, the authors propose a new diversity index of public health trainees. They posit that the diversity index may be used to compare the diversity of trainees across institutions. Although the proposed diversity index provides a starting point for examining diversity index across institutions, additional refinements may provide a more meaningful conceptualization and measurement of diversity as well as inclusivity of public health trainees entering the workforce.

First, in the words of Audre Lorde: "There is no thing as a single-issue struggle because we do not live single-issue lives." To heed this exhortation, recognizing and including multiple domains will help us fully capture the diversity of who we are and who we serve in future iterations of a diversity index of public health trainees.

This requires broadening and reconfiguring the conceptualization of a diversity index to be inclusive of dimensions such as: socioeconomic status, sexual orientation, biological sex and gender identity, geography, and disability status. A broadening and reconfiguration of such a diversity index does not dilute its power. Rather, it recognizes that all of these domains equally merit inclusion. And it means recognizing that racialized identity and ethnicity is one of many domains that interact and intersect with those also mentioned here to reflect the diversity and inclusivity of our population.

Second, the diversity of our public health trainees should continue to reflect the racial and ethnic diversity of the US. Although Asian Americans as a whole may not be underrepresented in the health professions, there is likely to be significant variation in representation across Asian American ethnicities among public health trainees. And these differences in representation intersect with key socioeconomic drivers, such as stark disparities in socioeconomic status, immigration status, linguistic and cultural differences, and experiences of anti-Asian racism and discrimination—factors that play significant roles in understanding the drivers of health inequalities across disaggregated Asian American ethnic groups. Furthermore, ensuring that there is and continues to be representation of Asian Americans among public health trainees can provide unique perspectives that would otherwise be missed in attempting to address the myriad health disparities among the multilingual and multicultural Asian American communities across the United States.

One final consideration is that our public health trainees at any given institution are from across the United States but also from around the world. Moreover, they may train in one geographic location and serve in another. How do we represent these trainees in a diversity index and what does this mean for a diversity index? Clearly, students coming from developing countries and from the global south enrich the diversity of our programs and help grow a global cadre of public health professionals. While their experiences of structural racism and discrimination and experience of inequities may be different from those of domestic students, their presence and inclusion recognizes that we need cross-cultural competency in order to promote health equity for populations across the world.

DIVERSITY IN WHAT WE TEACH

In addition to striving for intersectional diversity among our public health trainees, we require public health curricula that intentionally highlight the institutional and structural forces that undermine not only the public's health but also our public health mission. Importantly, public health trainees need to be able to apply this understanding to prioritize dismantling the barriers to equitable health care access and to create public health promotion and prevention strategies for health and well-being from a social justice perspective. Allowing trainees to think critically about the needs and assets of the diverse communities that they come from as well as those they intend to serve will allow more organic and meaningful engagement and public health action. Finally, training in leadership skills to meet the challenges of the complex forces that undermine population health is also a necessary component of training the next generation of public health faculty.[3,4]

CONCLUSIONS

Measuring diversity in the public health pipeline and the public health workforce is critical to successfully achieving the goals of our public health enterprise. The recent Supreme Court decision in *Students for Fair Admissions v President and Fellows of Harvard College* on June 29, 2023 (https://www.oyez.org/cases/2022/20-1199) dismantling affirmative action as currently constituted provides a moment for public health schools to reassess their admissions strategies to be even more inclusive. While we cannot ignore the centuries of educational, economic, and political inequality that have been directed at Black and Hispanic/Latino students in the United States, this moment may provide an opportunity for considering diversity across multiple domains—racialized identity, ethnicity, socioeconomic status, biological sex, gender identity, sexual orientation, geographic location, and disability status as they all matter. The health problems our populations face are complex and rooted in social, economic, and political systems established to sustain inequity. Promoting population health requires training and being trained by people who embody, understand, and have the lived experiences that allow us to dismantle the systems and structures that prevent us from attaining health for all. AJPH

CORRESPONDENCE

Correspondence should be sent to Farzana Kapadia, PhD, MPH, New York University, School of Global Public Health, 708 Broadway, Room 729, New York, NY 10003 (e-mail: farzana.kapadia@nyu.edu). Reprints can be ordered at http://www.ajph.org by clicking the "Reprints" link.

PUBLICATION INFORMATION

Full Citation: Kapadia F. Health equity requires public health workforce diversity and inclusivity: a public health of consequence, September 2023. *Am J Public Health*. 2023;113(9):936–938.

Acceptance Date: June 23, 2023.

DOI: https://doi.org/10.2105/AJPH.2023.307372

CONFLICTS OF INTEREST

The author has no conflicts of interest to disclose.

REFERENCES

1. Winslow C-EA, Park WH, Rosenau MJ, Welch WH, Turner CE. Report of the committee on public health training. *Am J Public Health*. 1923;13(10):837–841. https://doi.org/10.2105/AJPH.13.10.837
2. Krasna H, Fried L. Generation public health: fixing the broken bridge between public health education and the governmental workforce. *Am J Public Health*. 2021;111(8):1413–1417. https://doi.org/10.2105/AJPH.2021.306317
3. Koh HK. Educating future public health leaders. *Am J Public Health*. 2015;105(suppl 1):S11–S13. https://doi.org/10.2105/AJPH.2014.302385
4. Levy M, Gentry D, Klesges LM. Innovations in public health education: promoting professional development and a culture of health. *Am J Public Health*. 2015;105(suppl 1):S44–S45. https://doi.org/10.2105/AJPH.2014.302351

Hospital-Based Community Gardens as a Strategic Partner in Addressing Community Health Needs

Daniel R. George, PhD, MSc, and Amy E. Ethridge, MS, OTR/L

As part of community health needs assessments, US nonprofit hospitals are identifying a high prevalence of chronic diseases associated with poor diets. Institutions have responded by establishing nutrition-related initiatives such as farmers' markets and community gardens. There is public health value in demonstrating how these partnerships can help hospitals address identified community health needs. Here we describe diverse strategies undertaken by a hospital-based community garden at Penn State Milton S. Hershey Medical Center, explore implications for US hospitals, and provide implementation guidance. (*Am J Public Health*. 2023;113(9):939–942. https://doi.org/10.2105/AJPH.2023.307336)

AJPH September 2023, Vol 113, No. 9

The passage of the Affordable Care Act in 2010[1] has ushered in an era in which nonprofit hospitals must conduct community health needs assessments (CHNAs) and enact implementation plans to address identified needs. Failure to do so can result in loss of tax-exempt status and a financial penalty.[2] Given that institutional CHNAs are increasingly identifying a high prevalence of chronic diseases associated with poor diets (e.g., diabetes, cardiovascular disease, obesity[3]), there has been a trend toward hospitals supporting nutrition-related initiatives.[4] Previous research, for instance, has established the existence of more than 200 farmers' markets and community gardens associated with US hospitals,[5,6] as well as nearly 30 hospital-based organic farms involved in food production.[7]

There is a need to disseminate strategies demonstrating how such organizational partnerships can help hospitals pursue CHNA goals. Here we offer a descriptive overview of dynamic programs emerging from a hospital-based community garden at Penn State Milton S. Hershey Medical Center to address extant community health needs. In addition, we provide an implementation guide (available as a supplement to the online version of this article at http://www.ajph.org).

INTERVENTION AND IMPLEMENTATION

Our hospital-based community garden was established in 2014, shortly after the institution's first CHNA identified high rates of obesity, cardiovascular disease, and diabetes as well as prevalent psychosocial issues (e.g., loneliness and isolation). Its primary purpose was to offer plots to community members, employees, students, clinical groups, and local nonprofits to engage in healthy food production, reduce chronic disease, and build community bonds. Institutional leadership committed a one-acre space in a former construction staging area, and community volunteers built 125 raised-bed plots. Initial infrastructure included hoses, rain collection cisterns, composting pits, benches, gazebos, picnic tables, and an eight-foot-high fence.

A portion of the garden was devoted to philanthropic purposes, with produce donated to food-insecure community members. The garden was promoted through the hospital's strategic services and local media. In 2017, in response to high community demand, the garden expanded to two acres and 234 plots (Figure 1).

PLACE, TIME, AND PERSONS

The garden operates during March through November and is run as a nonprofit with a governing board. A part-time manager funded by corporate sponsorships, grants, and private donations provides day-to-day garden a

b

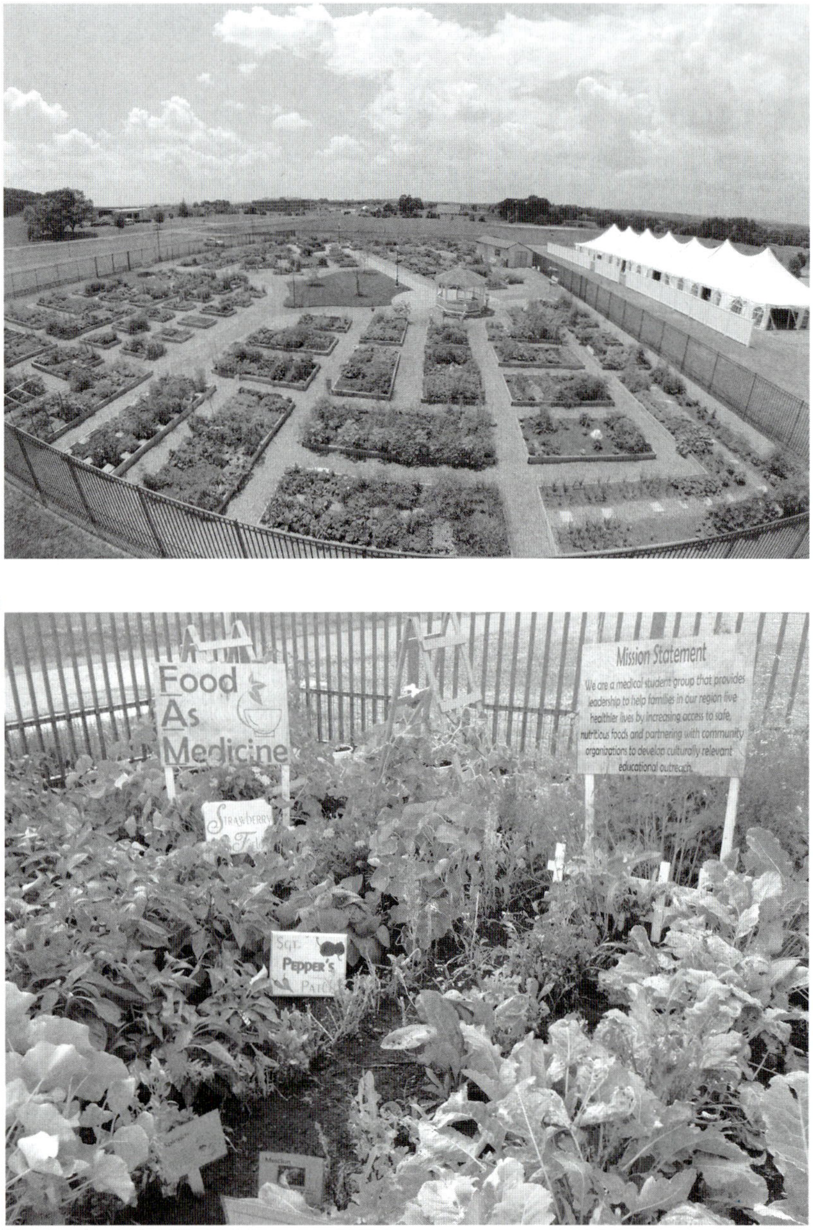

FIGURE 1— The Penn State Milton S. Hershey Medical Center Community Garden Includes (a) 234 Plots in a Two-Acre Space and (b) a Variety of Nutrition-Oriented Initiatives in the Medical Student–Led Food as Medicine Plot

oversight. Gardeners receive plots on a first-come, first-served basis with a $45 suggested donation. Tools are provided, and ground rules set collective expectations (e.g., gardeners must use organic methods and pull weeds). Plots are overseen by community members, faculty, clinical staff, graduate students, and charitable organizations.

PURPOSE

We sought to use our hospital-based community garden to encourage healthy food production and facilitate innovative programming to address chronic disease and other local health needs (e.g., loneliness and isolation) identified through the CHNA.

EVALUATION AND ADVERSE EFFECTS

Over a decade, the garden has fostered diverse initiatives serving various identified needs as part of the hospital's CHNA and has also evolved to address other areas (Table 1):

- Charitable plots in the garden have produced annual averages of 2800 pounds of produce donations for local food banks to distribute to food-insecure community members. The plots have also generated donations of cut flowers to various community groups (e.g., Meals on Wheels, retirement homes). Gardeners make weekly donations, weighing and recording their weekly contributions using an on-site scale.
- A Food as Medicine initiative led by medical students has used a 400-square-foot plot to address food insecurity and nutrition education.[8,9] Students partnered with the hospital's driving instructor to transport weekly produce donations to migrant workers living in food deserts. More recently, produce has been donated to food-insecure refugee families resettled in central Pennsylvania. In response to a high overweight rate for children in the hospital's service area (33.4%),[10] students have also used the plot to provide education on healthy eating for elementary school students. Anecdotally, students have viewed the plot as a resource for self-care and burnout mitigation during medical school.[8]

TABLE 1— Penn State Milton S. Hershey Medical Center Community Garden Programs and Objectives

Program	Objective(s)
Charitable plots	Generate produce donations for local food banks to distribute to food-insecure community members
Food as Medicine	Empower medical students to grow produce and provide nutrition education for food-insecure families and at-risk populations (e.g., recently resettled refugees)
Prescription Produce	Allow clinicians to refer patients (e.g., young adult cancer survivors and adults at risk for cardiovascular disease) to a program pairing them with local master gardeners to learn how to cultivate and prepare healthy foods
Eating disorder recovery	Enable occupational therapists to engage patients living with eating disorders in horticulture therapy and cultivation of produce for use in a clinic food preparation group
Skin cancer prevention	Provide free sunscreen dispensers from the dermatology clinic to promote healthy skin care and grow cruciferous vegetables for research in treating melanoma
Hospital cafeteria food production	Establish a venue for chefs to grow herbs and vegetables for food preparation and integrate produce into cafeteria and inpatient menus
Inclusive design components	Facilitate the participation of elderly and differently abled community members via inclusive design elements (e.g., wheelchair accessibility and waist-high raised beds)
Medicinal plant plot	Cultivate plants used in folk and traditional medicine and pharmaceutical development and provide community education for local students interested in health care careers
Composting partnerships	Forge partnerships between the garden and hospital food services to divert organic waste from the cafeteria to the garden compost pit
Garden pollination	Establish beehive colonies in proximity to the garden and increase native plants and wildflowers on the hospital campus

- Research faculty committed to chronic disease reduction partnered with clinicians in the Cancer Institute and Family and Community Medicine to engage at-risk patients in healthier eating patterns via the garden. Specifically, the Prescription Produce initiative enabled clinicians to "prescribe" young adult cancer survivors a garden plot and pair them with local master gardeners to learn how to cultivate and prepare healthy foods over a growing season. Subsequent initiatives have engaged patients at risk for cardiovascular disease. Both programs have shown preliminary benefits for patients (i.e., increased dietary intake of produce, physical activity, and quality of life).[11,12]
- An Eating Disorders Clinic occupational therapist has used a plot for horticulture therapy as well as growing produce for use in the clinic. Garden field trips occur after mealtime groups for stress management purposes. Cultivated produce has been used in the clinic kitchen to help patients practice food preparation skills and follow prescription meal plans.
- In response to rising local skin cancer rates,[11] the dermatology department has provided free sunscreen dispensers to promote healthy skin care. Department faculty have also grown cruciferous vegetables rich in a class of molecules known as isothiocyanates, which can inhibit a key signaling pathway for melanoma cell survival, and studied the efficacy of extracted compounds in treating melanoma.
- Hospital executive chefs have cultivated a plot growing herbs for food preparation and integrated produce into cafeteria and inpatient menus.
- The garden is wheelchair accessible and has seven waist-high beds to facilitate the participation of elderly and differently abled community members in cultivation of healthier lifestyles.
- A medicinal plant plot tended by a bench scientist has grown dozens of species of plants used in folk and traditional medicine and pharmaceutical development.[8] This space has been used for community education with local students interested in health care careers.
- A medical student developed a composting partnership with hospital food services that diverted 220 pounds of organic food waste from the cafeteria to the garden compost pit each week.
- Hospital employees established five beehive colonies in proximity to the garden and advocated for the institution to replace mowed turf grass with native plants and wildflowers.

Adverse effects have been negligible but have included increases in campus traffic, maintenance responsibilities, and costs (e.g., liability insurance).

SUSTAINABILITY

The garden is entering its 10th season with a substantial waiting list for plots. Funding has been secure, and consistent management has helped maintain organizational continuity and adherence to governing principles. The hospital documents yearly achievements as part of its CHNA and highlights the garden and its programs in annual reports. Taken together, the initiatives described here have resulted in modest preliminary benefits for at-risk patients, community members, and students,[8–12] as well as generating grant funding and scholarship for faculty and students and catalyzing programs in service of education and environmental health. The hospital is exploring converting 10 acres of additional land into an organic farm in partnership with the Rodale Institute, a nonprofit that supports organic farming.

PUBLIC HEALTH SIGNIFICANCE

This case study demonstrates how a hospital's CHNA process can guide institutional investments in infrastructure such as community gardens that become dynamic spaces in support of local health promotion. If smaller hospitals lack space for gardening infrastructure, they may nonetheless find it useful to partner with existing community gardens. Our experience suggests that public health ingenuity can emerge organically from an initiative such as a community garden; in other words, a hospital does not have to fully drive or fund all programming benefiting community health but, rather, can establish or align with existing gardening space and unleash the creativity of employees, community members, and organizations around CHNA goals. Moreover, supply chain issues during the COVID-19 pandemic have underscored the benefits of local food production as a component of healthier, more resilient communities.

Although limited to a single institution, our experience establishes strategies that other hospital-based gardens can use in dynamically addressing community health needs. Future researchers can establish broader trends, patterns, and best practices across existing hospital-based gardens, farmers' markets, and farms. AJPH

ABOUT THE AUTHORS

Daniel R. George is with the Department of Humanities and Public Health Sciences, Penn State College of Medicine, Hershey, PA. Amy E. Ethridge is with the Eating Disorders Clinic, Penn State Milton S. Hershey Medical Center, Hershey, PA.

CORRESPONDENCE

Correspondence should be sent to Daniel R. George, PhD, MSc, 500 University Dr, Penn State College of Medicine, Hershey, PA 17033 (e-mail: dgeorge1@pennstatehealth.psu.edu). Reprints can be ordered at http://www.ajph.org by clicking the "Reprints" link.

PUBLICATION INFORMATION

Full Citation: George DR, Ethridge AE. Hospital-based community gardens as a strategic partner in addressing community health needs. *Am J Public Health*. 2023;113(9):939–942.

Acceptance Date: May 11, 2023.

DOI: https://doi.org/10.2105/AJPH.2023.307336

CONTRIBUTORS

The authors were equally responsible for writing, reviewing, and editing the article.

CONFLICTS OF INTEREST

The authors report no conflicts of interest.

HUMAN PARTICIPANT PROTECTION

No human research participants were directly involved in this work.

REFERENCES

1. Patient Protection and Affordable Care Act, Section 9007. Available at: http://www.gpo.gov/fdsys/pkg/BILLS-111hr3590enr/pdf/BILLS-111hr3590enr.pdf. Accessed January 19, 2023.
2. Young GJ, Chou CH, Alexander J, Lee SYD, Raver E. Provision of community benefits by tax-exempt US hospitals. *N Engl J Med*. 2013;368(16):1519–1527. https://doi.org/10.1056/NEJMsa1210239
3. Gunja MZ, Gumas ED, Williams RD. US health care from a global perspective, 2022: accelerating spending, worsening outcomes. Available at: https://www.commonwealthfund.org/publications/issue-briefs/2023/jan/us-health-care-global-perspective-2022. Accessed January 19, 2023.
4. George DR, Rovniak L, Snyder G. The role of nutrition-related initiatives in addressing community health needs assessments. *Am J Health Educ*. 2017;48(1):58–63. https://doi.org/10.1080/19325037.2016.1250019
5. George DR, Kraschnewski JL, Rovniak LS. Public health potential of farmers' markets on medical center campuses: a case study from Penn State Milton S. Hershey Medical Center. *Am J Public Health*. 2011;101(12):2226–2232. https://doi.org/10.2105/AJPH.2011.300197 https://ajph.aphapublications.org/doi/full/10.2105/AJPH.2011.300197
6. George DR, Kraschnewski J, Rovniak L, Hanson R. Sciamanna C. A growing opportunity: community gardens associated with US hospitals and academic health centers. *Prev Med Rep*. 2015;2:35–39. https://doi.org/10.1016/j.pmedr.2014.12.003
7. Veldheer S, George DR. Strategies to help healthcare organizations execute their food system leadership responsibilities. *AMA J Ethics*. 2022;24(10):E994–E1003. https://doi.org/10.1001/amajethics.2022.994
8. George DR, Hanson R, Gilman F, Edris W. Medicinal plants—the next generation. *Lancet*. 2016;387(10015):220–221. https://doi.org/10.1016/S0140-6736(16)00052-0
9. George DR, Manglani M, Minnehan K, et al. Examining feasibility of mentoring families at a farmers' market and community garden. *Am J Health Educ*. 2016;47(2):94–98. https://doi.org/10.1080/19325037.2015.1133340
10. Penn State Milton S. Hershey Medical Center. A five-county regional community health needs assessment. Available at: https://ppimhs.org/wp-content/uploads/2021/10/2016_CHNA_Five-County_Implementation_Strategy.pdf. Accessed May 3, 2023.
11. Winkels RM, Artrip R, Tupinio M, Veldheer S, Dandekar S, George DR. Opportunities for growth: a community gardening pilot intervention pairing adolescent and young adult cancer survivors with master gardeners. *J Adolesc Young Adult Oncol*. 2020;9(1):115–119. https://doi.org/10.1089/jayao.2019.0035
12. Veldheer S, Winkels RM, Cooper J, et al. Growing healthy hearts: gardening program feasibility in a hospital-based community garden. *J Nutr Educ Behav*. 2020;52(10):958–963. https://doi.org/10.1016/j.jneb.2020.07.006

A Mortality Surveillance Collaboration Between a Health System and Public Health Department

Scott A. Simpson, MD, MPH, Ryan Loh, PhD, Laura Elliott, MA, Rachel Everhart, PhD, Conlin Bass, MPH, Kirk Bol, MSPH, Steve Boylls, and Laura Podewils, PhD

We describe a collaboration between a health system and public health department to create a mortality surveillance system. The collaboration enabled the health system to identify more than six times the number of deaths identified through local system medical records alone. This powerful epidemiological process, combining the nuanced data captured through clinical care in health systems with subsequent data on mortality, drives quality improvement, scientific research, and epidemiology that can be of particular benefit to underserved communities. (*Am J Public Health*. 2023;113(9):943–946. https://doi.org/10.2105/AJPH.2023.307335)

AJPH September 2023, Vol 113, No. 9

Identifying patient death after discharge is elemental to improving treatment in health systems. Here we describe a collaboration between the Colorado Department of Public Health and Environment (CDPHE) and the Denver Health and Hospital Authority (DH) to implement a mortality surveillance system in support of clinical operations, quality improvement, and research.

INTERVENTION AND IMPLEMENTATION

Every quarter, DH transmits information on patients served to the CDPHE Vital Statistics Program. CDPHE uses a matching algorithm to match DH patients to state mortality data. Mortality data are returned to DH and stored in an enterprise data warehouse. Figure A (available as a supplement to the online version of this article at http://www.ajph.org) illustrates the matching process, key personnel, and data elements involved. CDPHE's interstate compacts allow ascertainment of out-of-state deaths, and a bilateral data use agreement governs the collaboration. Facts of death (e.g., date and time) are available to the health system within days, whereas manner of death (e.g., suicide) and cause of death (illness or injury) are available within months. All patients with a medical record (approximately 1.7 million individuals) are matched each quarter to ensure that delayed or updated mortality reports are included.

PLACE, TIME, AND PERSONS

DH is an integrated academic health care system that serves the city and county of Denver, Colorado. DH's services include an acute care hospital, a level 1 adult trauma center, a level 2 pediatric trauma center, 10 federally qualified health centers, 19 school-based health centers, behavioral health services, a 911 emergency response system, correctional care services, and the Public Health Institute at Denver Health. The described implementation includes all DH patients since April 2016 with a medical record (Table 1).

PURPOSE

This public health practice program uses vital statistics data for ongoing clinical and public health operations, quality improvement, and scientific research. The collaboration began with an effort to identify risk factors for death by suicide after emergency department care. Much suicide prevention research relies on smaller clinical trials that may not reflect real-world practice or include certain patient populations such as those who are homeless, incarcerated, or of minority race/ethnicity.[1] Initially, we conducted a 27-month study to better ascertain suicide deaths, which are of infrequent incidence. The results revealed significant limitations in existing approaches to emergency department–based suicide screening.[2,3]

TABLE 1— Characteristics of Patients in the Mortality Surveillance System: Denver, CO, 2016–2023

Characteristic	Unduplicated DH Patients, No. (%)	Deaths Identified in Local DH System, No. (%)	Additional Unduplicated Deaths Identified From CDPHE, No. (%)
Total	1 721 554	11 972	72 875
Female	797 726 (46.3)	4 415 (36.9)	27 643 (37.9)
Race/ethnicity			
Non-Hispanic Black/African American	135 443 (7.9)	1 507 (12.6)	6 130 (8.4)
Hispanic	445 017 (25.8)	3 918 (32.7)	11 795 (16.2)
Non-Hispanic White	553 280 (32.1)	4 351 (36.3)	26 291 (36.1)
Missing/other	587 814 (34.1)	2 196 (18.3)	28 659 (39.3)
Ever homeless	64 552 (3.7)	804 (6.7)	5 091 (7.0)
Manner of death[a]			
Natural	61 742 (72.8)	6 021 (50.3)	55 721 (76.5)
Suicide	3 515 (4.1)	229 (1.9)	3 286 (4.5)
External cause[b]	13 349 (15.7)	1 659 (13.9)	11 690 (16.0)
Missing/unknown/other	6 241 (7.4)	4 063 (33.9)	2 178 (3.0)

Note. CDPHE = Colorado Department of Public Health and Environment; DH = Denver Health.
Source. Data are based on Denver Health medical records from April 2016 to January 10, 2023.
[a]The percentages for manner of death among unduplicated DH patients are based on the total number of deaths identified in the local DH system plus additional unduplicated deaths identified from CDPHE (n = 84 847).
[b]Including accidental trauma, homicide, and overdose.[2]

We then sought to match mortality data regularly for operational efforts. A 2018 grant to CDPHE funded technical expertise to conduct regular data exchanges. A standing data exchange agreement was formalized, and technical processes were refined. For example, matching algorithms were improved and standard work incorporated iterative matches to reduce the likelihood of reclassifications being missed.[4]

The final and current state of the implementation was further motivated by the COVID-19 pandemic. In 2021, DH began outreach efforts with patients to schedule vaccinations. However, a significant number of elderly patients were found to be deceased. Attempting to contact these individuals was a distraction of limited resources and often resulted in distressing interactions for familial survivors and staff. DH then had to identify all patients with a medical record who were deceased.

EVALUATION AND ADVERSE EFFECTS

Before matching with state data, DH identified 11 972 patients as deceased among those since 2016 with a medical record (Table 1). An additional 72 875 deceased patients were identified after matching with CDPHE. Consistent with previous years, not all patients identified as deceased in the local DH medical record could be matched to the CDPHE mortality data.[5] Among the 11 972 deceased individuals identified in DH records, matching rates with CDPHE were higher for those with than without an encounter since 2016, when a new electronic medical record was implemented (87% versus 38%). Deaths among DH patients with only an emergency department encounter were matched to CDPHE data 88% of the time, and matching increased to 95% if patients were also hospitalized and had an outpatient encounter.

Systematic limitations in identifying deceased patients pose a challenge in application of these data. Patients who are not identified as deceased are presumed alive in most evaluation and research activities. Thus, patient populations that are less likely to be matched are at greater risk of underreported mortality. Poor capture of demographic data may be more common among individuals who are experiencing homelessness or have substance use disorders.[6] Death certificate data for gender nonbinary individuals include only legal sex, whereas DH medical records allow patients to provide both sex and gender identification. No gold standard for matching exists.[6,7] Standardization of data collection and reporting across health care and public health systems would mitigate these limitations; multiple encounters in a health system may also improve the quality of demographic data and ability to match.

SUSTAINABILITY

This public health collaboration has been permanently operationalized by both parties consistent with CDPHE's vision for a "healthy and sustainable Colorado" and DH's role as a learning health system, which is "a health system in which internal data and experience are systematically integrated with external evidence, and that knowledge is put into practice."[8] Learning health system activities are financially incentivized by private and public payors and reductions in the cost of provided care. The collaboration has also supported awards of competitive external funding.

PUBLIC HEALTH SIGNIFICANCE

This collaboration exemplifies how health systems and public health practitioners can partner to deliver better health care. For the health system, the ready availability of mortality outcomes drives quality improvement and research efforts. This information enables systematic review of individual outcomes (e.g., debriefings with providers whose patients die by suicide). Figure A illustrates data distribution and review processes within the health system.

This work is particularly notable for its promise to reflect underserved communities in public health programming and effectiveness studies. Research involving such population-level data can incorporate clinical interventions among more heterogeneous populations than is the case in clinical trials.[9] DH applies these data in emphasizing programs that address a range of behavioral emergencies and health concerns among underserved populations.[10,11]

The public health department uses these data for program planning and policymaking. For example, CDPHE expanded a telephonic outreach program for patients at high risk of suicide to include individuals with recent nonsuicidal overdoses after data demonstrated high overdose mortality among patients with an emergency department presentation for psychiatric care.[11] Although no single data system will capture the totality and nuances of a patient's lived experience, health systems routinely maintain rich individualized data for delivering clinical care.

The approach described here has advantages over previously described efforts. Matching mortality data with regional health information exchanges would capture larger populations. However, health information exchanges are expensive, may be technically limited in matching patients, and require cooperation among multiple institutions to improve data capture and matching.[12] The described bilateral partnership is financially sustainable, has minimal reporting delay and so can be used for iterative quality improvement, and can be recurrently optimized to improve matching processes. Moreover, as health systems expand in size and their records come to include large regional areas, these systems must become key partners in efforts to improve population mortality.

The mortality surveillance system described here thus stands to inform clinicians' individual practice, better represent underserved communities in health innovation, and direct resources to high-risk patients. AJPH

ABOUT THE AUTHORS

Scott Simpson, Ryan Loh, Laura Elliott, Rachel Everhart, and Laura Podewils are with the Denver Health and Hospital Authority, Denver, CO. Conlin Bass, Kirk Bol, and Steve Boylls are with the Colorado Department of Public Health and Environment, Denver.

CORRESPONDENCE

Correspondence should be sent to Scott Simpson, MD, MPH, Denver Health, 777 Bannock St MC 0116, Denver, CO 80204 (e-mail: scott.simpson@dhha.org). Reprints can be ordered at http://www.ajph.org by clicking the "Reprints" link.

PUBLICATION INFORMATION

Full Citation: Simpson SA, Loh R, Elliott L, et al. A mortality surveillance collaboration between a health system and public health department. *Am J Public Health*. 2023;113(9):943–946.

Acceptance Date: May 11, 2023.

DOI: https://doi.org/10.2105/AJPH.2023.307335

CONTRIBUTORS

S. A. Simpson was the lead author. R. Loh, C. Bass, K. Bol, and L. Podewils assisted substantively in drafting and revising. S. A. Simpson, R. Loh, L. Elliott, R. Everhart, K. Bol, S. Boylls, and L. Podewils conceived and designed the analyses. S. A. Simpson, R. Loh, R. Everhart, C. Bass, K. Bol, and L. Podewils conceived and led the implementation of the program. R. Loh, L. Elliott, K. Bol, S. Boylls, and L. Podewils collected the data, performed analyses, and implemented key elements of the program. All of the authors edited the final version of the article.

ACKNOWLEDGMENTS

This article describes work that was supported by multiple sources, including grant R18HS027389 awarded to Denver Health by the Agency for Healthcare Research and Quality and grant H79SM080284 awarded to the Colorado Department of Public Health and Environment by the Substance Abuse and Mental Health Services Administration.

Note. The content is solely the responsibility of the authors and does not necessarily represent the official views of the sponsoring or authors' employing agencies.

CONFLICTS OF INTEREST

The authors have no potential or actual conflicts of interest to disclose.

HUMAN PARTICIPANT PROTECTION

This study was authorized by the Colorado Multiple Institutional Review Board with a waiver of informed consent.

REFERENCES

1. Simpson SA, Loh RM, Goans CRR. New data on suicide risk assessment in the emergency department reveal the need for new approaches in research and clinical practice. *Psychol Med*. 2023;53(3):1122–1123. https://doi.org/10.1017/S0033291721001653
2. Simpson SA, Goans C, Loh R, Ryall K, Middleton MCA, Dalton A. Suicidal ideation is insensitive to suicide risk after emergency department discharge: performance characteristics of the

Columbia-Suicide Severity Rating Scale Screener. *Acad Emerg Med.* 2021;28(6):621–629. https://doi.org/10.1111/acem.14198

3. Simpson SA, Goans CRR, Loh RM, Ryall KA, Middleton M, Dalton A. Use of an agitation measure to screen for suicide and self-harm risk among emergency department patients. *J Acad Consult Liaison Psychiatry.* 2023;64(1):3–12. https://doi.org/10.1016/j.jaclp.2022.07.004
4. Education Development Center. Zero suicide. Available at: https://zerosuicide.edc.org. Accessed January 6, 2023.
5. Conway RBN, Armistead MG, Denney MJ, Smith GS. Validating the matching of patients in the linkage of a large hospital system's EHR with state and national death databases. *Appl Clin Inform.* 2021;12(1):82–89. https://doi.org/10.1055/s-0040-1722220
6. Ferris LM, Weiner JP, Saloner B, Kharrazi H. Comparing person-level matching algorithms to identify risk across disparate datasets among patients with a controlled substance prescription: retrospective analysis. *JAMA Open.* 2022;5(1):ooac020. https://doi.org/10.1093/jamiaopen/ooac020
7. Godlove T, Ball AW. Patient matching within a health information exchange. *Perspect Health Inf Manag.* 2015;12:1g.
8. Bindman A. How learning health systems learn: lessons from the field. Available at: https://www.ahrq.gov/sites/default/files/wysiwyg/lhs/how_learning_health_systems_learn.pdf. Accessed May 1, 2023.
9. Ma MA, Gutierrez DE, Frausto JM, Al-Delaimy WK. Minority representation in clinical trials in the United States: trends over the past 25 years. *Mayo Clin Proc.* 2021;96(1):264–266. https://doi.org/10.1016/j.mayocp.2020.10.027
10. Casher GA, Sutton B, Roosevelt G, Simpson SA. Evaluation of an integrated psychology service in a pediatric emergency department and urgent care. *Pediatr Emerg Care.* 2022;38(2):e697–e702. https://doi.org/10.1097/PEC.0000000000002328
11. Simpson SA, Shy BD, Loh RM. More than suicide: mortality after emergency psychiatric care and implications for practice. *J Acad Consult Liaison Psychiatry.* 2022;63(4):354–362. https://doi.org/10.1016/j.jaclp.2021.12.009
12. Devine EB, Totten AM, Gorman P, et al. Health information exchange use (1990–2015): a systematic review. *EGEMS (Wash DC).* 2017;5(1):27. https://doi.org/10.5334/egems.249

Timely Second-Dose Completion of mRNA COVID-19 Vaccination at Community-Based and Mobile Vaccine Clinics in Maryland

Cassandra Parent, BSc, Benjamin F. Bigelow, MD, Stephen D. Sisson, MD, Diego Martínez, PhD, Cui Yang, PhD, and Kathleen R. Page, MD

To assess factors associated with timely second-dose completion, we analyzed COVID-19 vaccine data from community-based and mobile vaccine clinics in Maryland. Overall, 85.3% of patients received a timely second dose. Factors associated with a timely second dose included Latino ethnicity (adjusted odds ratio [AOR] = 1.5; 95% confidence interval [CI] = 1.1, 2.0) and receipt of the first dose at community-based vaccine clinics (AOR = 2.1; 95% CI = 1.8, 2.5). Future health initiatives for underserved communities should focus on establishing vaccine clinics in trusted community spaces with culturally sensitive support. (*Am J Public Health*. 2023;113(9):947–951. https://doi.org/10.2105/AJPH.2023.307338)

AJPH September 2023, Vol 113, No. 9

The COVID-19 pandemic has disproportionately affected minoritized groups. As of August 2022, age-adjusted cumulative COVID-19 death rates were twice as high among Latino and Black patients than White patients.[1] Within Latino communities, undocumented immigrants and those with limited English proficiency face language barriers, concerns about immigration status, stigma, lack of trust, and difficulty navigating the medical system.[2,3]

INTERVENTION AND IMPLEMENTATION

To address disparities faced by Latino immigrants, a coalition was established between the Johns Hopkins Health System (JHHS), religious leaders, and community-based organizations to promote COVID-19 vaccinations.[4,5] Vaccines were delivered at a local church (Sacred Heart) and in a mobile clinic.

Vaccine clinics at Sacred Heart were held consistently every Wednesday and Friday between 4 PM and 7 PM, except for holidays. Mobile clinic locations were determined by the local health department, local leaders, community outreach workers, and the request of community organizations. Most sites were visited three to four times. Between April 27 and August 31, 2021, all patients vaccinated at Sacred Heart received a phone call from bilingual health workers to remind them about their second-dose appointment. Starting on September 1, 2021, all patients vaccinated at Sacred Heart and a subgroup of patients vaccinated in other mobile clinics received mobile phone short message service (SMS) reminders from bicultural and bilingual community health workers through a Health Insurance Portability and Accountability Act (HIPAA)-compliant SMS platform, WelTel, about their follow-up dose.[6]

At the time of vaccination, demographic information about the patient (including race, ethnicity, and gender) was collected, as well as information about any previous COVID-19 doses. Vaccine administration was recorded in the JHHS electronic medical record (EMR) system and reported to the state of Maryland. On a weekly basis, the EMR system checks for updated vaccination information on patients within the JHHS and updates patients' records if they received additional doses from nonaffiliated sites.

PLACE, TIME, AND PERSONS

Patients who were vaccinated at Sacred Heart or a mobile clinic through JHHS and received their first dose between April 27, 2021 and April 21, 2022 were included in the current analysis. We excluded patients vaccinated before April 27, 2021, because vaccine availability was limited prior to this date and allocated only to certain high-risk individuals. All JHHS employees and Johns Hopkins students were excluded, as full vaccination was a mandatory requirement for employment and enrollment and thus was not representative of the general public. Patients younger than 16 years were also excluded because of limited vaccine eligibility during a large portion of this study period. Finally, patients who received the Johnson & Johnson vaccine were excluded because only one dose was recommended during the study period. We categorized vaccination timing as before or after September 1, 2021, because of the launch of WelTel messaging and the start of many statewide vaccination recommendations.[7]

PURPOSE

An initial course of two doses of the Moderna or Pfizer/BioNTech vaccine followed by subsequent booster doses remains essential for reducing poor COVID-19 outcomes.[8,9] However, a study examining more than 150 million American patients between December 14, 2020 and December 31, 2021 found that Latino patients were more likely to have a missed second dose than White patients.[10] To address these disparities, we assessed the factors associated with timely second-dose completion at the JHHS community vaccination initiative. The results can be used to inform future vaccine programs for vulnerable populations.

EVALUATION AND ADVERSE EFFECTS

Unadjusted and adjusted odds ratios were calculated to determine which patient factors were associated with timely second-dose completion. Timely second-dose completion was defined

TABLE 1— Characteristics of Patients and Factors Associated With Completion of a Second Dose of COVID-19 Vaccine: Maryland, April 2021–April 2022

Characteristics	Total	Completed Second Dose, No. (%)	OR (95% CI)	AOR[a] (95% CI)
Age, y				
16–25	1981	1669 (84.3)	1 (Ref)	1 (Ref)
26–44	3681	3120 (84.8)	1.0 (0.9, 1.2)	1.0 (0.9, 1.2)
45–64	1610	1412 (87.7)	1.3 (1.1, 1.6)	1.3 (1.0, 1.5)
≥ 65	246	209 (85.0)	1.0 (0.7, 1.5)	1.3 (0.9, 2.0)
Gender[b]				
Male	4205	3509 (83.4)	1 (Ref)	1 (Ref)
Female	3313	2901 (87.6)	1.4 (1.2, 1.6)	1.1 (1.0, 1.3)
Race/ethnicity				
Non-Latino White	291	230 (79.0)	1 (Ref)	1 (Ref)
Non-Latino Black	960	799 (83.2)	1.3 (1.0, 1.8)	1.2 (0.9, 1.7)
Latino	5873	5150 (87.7)	1.9 (1.4, 2.5)	1.5 (1.1, 2.0)
Asian	178	50 (28.1)	0.1 (0.1, 0.2)	0.3 (0.2, 0.5)
Other	216	181 (83.8)	1.4 (0.9, 2.2)	0.9 (0.5, 1.3)
Vaccination location				
Mobile clinic	2456	1705 (69.4)	1 (Ref)	1 (Ref)
Sacred Heart	5062	4386 (86.6)	2.9 (2.5, 3.2)	2.1 (1.8, 2.5)
Vaccination timing				
On or before Sep 1, 2021	4883	4445 (91.0)	1 (Ref)	1 (Ref)
After Sep 1, 2021	2635	1646 (62.5)	0.2 (0.1, 0.2)	0.2 (0.2, 0.2)
Type of vaccine				
Moderna	229	146 (63.8)	1 (Ref)	1 (Ref)
Pfizer	7289	6264 (85.9)	3.5 (2.6, 4.6)	1.8 (1.2, 2.5)

Note. AOR = adjusted odds ratio; CI = confidence interval; OR = odds ratio. The total number of patients was 7518.

[a]Adjusted for all variables.
[b]Five patients of unknown gender were excluded here, and all five got both doses.

as receiving the second dose within six weeks after the first dose. Covariates were chosen on the basis of data availability and included age, gender, race/ethnicity, location of dose, timing of dose, and type of vaccine. Patients self-reported their race/ethnicity from a set of categories, including non-Latino White, non-Latino Black, Latino, Asian, and other. Odds ratios were calculated with a 95% confidence interval, and statistical significance was determined by a two-sided *P* value of less than .05.

There was a total of 7518 patients included in the final analysis, with 6410 (85.3%) receiving at least two doses. Table 1 presents the characteristics of the patients and the factors associated with timely second-dose completion. Patients aged 45 to 64 years were more likely to receive a timely second dose (adjusted odds ratio [AOR] = 1.3; 95% confidence interval [CI] = 1.0, 1.5). Latinos were significantly more likely to get a timely second dose than Whites (AOR = 1.5; 95% CI = 1.1, 2.0), and Asians were the least likely to receive a timely second dose (AOR = 0.3; 95% CI = 0.2, 0.5).

Patients who received their first dose at Sacred Heart were significantly more likely to get their second dose within six weeks than patients who received their first dose from the mobile clinic (AOR = 2.1; 95% CI = 1.8, 2.5). Patients who were vaccinated after September 1, 2021 were significantly less likely to receive both doses (AOR = 0.2; 95% CI = 0.2, 0.2). Similar findings are presented in Figure 1, with second-dose completion rates at both sites decreasing over time. Patients who received the Pfizer/BioNTech vaccine were also significantly more likely to receive a second dose than their Moderna counterparts (AOR = 1.8; 95% CI = 1.2, 2.5), but this could be associated with timing, as Moderna was frequently used early in the vaccination campaign. This analysis is limited by variations during the intervention, such as differences in vaccination reminders, and may not be generalizable to other minoritized communities.

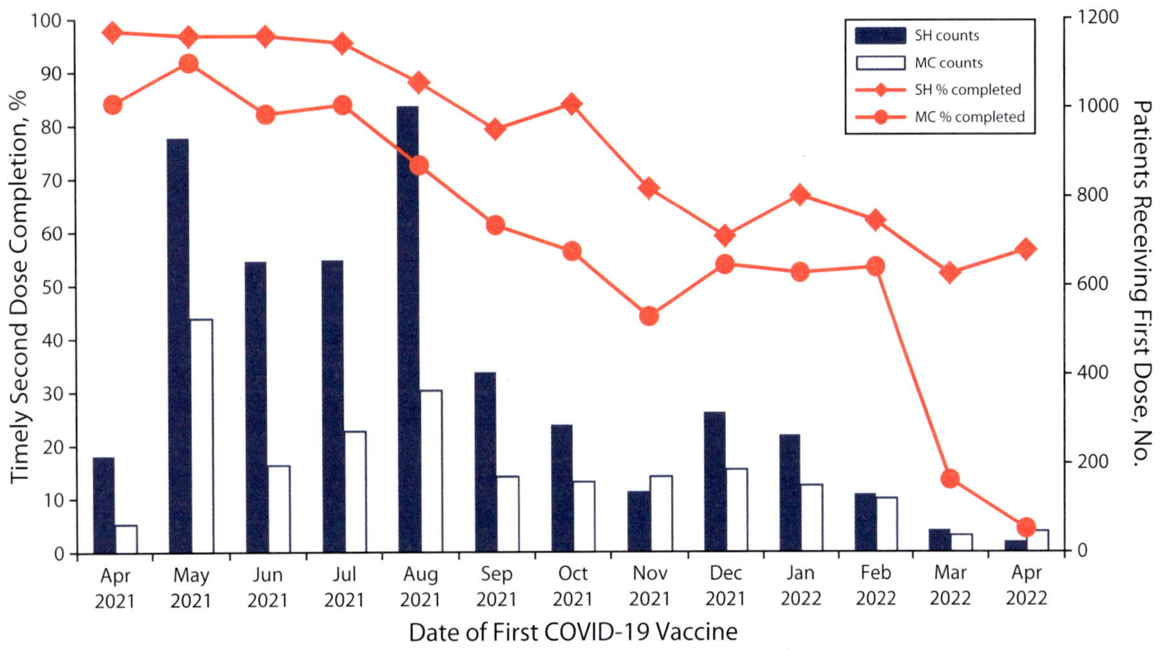

	Apr 2021	May 2021	Jun 2021	Jul 2021	Aug 2021	Sep 2021	Oct 2021	Nov 2021	Dec 2021	Jan 2022	Feb 2022	Mar 2022	Apr 2022
SH counts	217	932	654	657	1003	404	285	135	313	262	129	48	23
MC counts	63	526	196	272	363	170	158	170	186	149	120	37	46
SH % completed	97.7	96.8	96.8	95.4	88	79.2	83.9	68.1	59.1	66.8	62	52.1	56.5
MC % completed	84.1	91.8	82.1	83.8	72.5	61.2	56.3	44.1	53.8	52.3	53.3	13.5	4.3

FIGURE 1— Timely Completion of a Second Dose of COVID-19 Vaccine Over Time, Stratified by Location: Maryland, April 2021–April 2022

Note. MC = mobile clinic; SH = Sacred Heart (a local church). The total number of patients was 7518.

SUSTAINABILITY

Community-based and mobile vaccine clinics achieved a high second-dose completion rate. The coalition with community partners and a strong workforce of bilingual community health workers provided critical insights into intervention implementation facilitators and helped to identify barriers to building a foundation for COVID-19 and other vaccine equity initiatives. Additionally, the methods used in this intervention could be sustained through adaptation in other health services.

PUBLIC HEALTH SIGNIFICANCE

Patients who were vaccinated at a local church were significantly more likely to have a timely second-dose completion compared with those vaccinated at mobile clinics. This highlights the importance of collaborating with trusted community-based partners for public health interventions. Compared with mobile clinics, the schedule at the church was very consistent over time, which likely also facilitated second-dose completion.

Among racial groups, Latino patients had the highest timely second-dose completion rate (87.7%) and were more likely to receive a second dose than Whites after controlling for other covariates. In contrast, nationwide statistics show that Latino patients have lower rates of second-dose completion than their White counterparts.[10] Our findings may reflect the benefits of implementing free and culturally competent services at trusted, convenient, and accessible places for the community. Bilingual and secure SMS vaccine reminders from community health workers may have also contributed to high completion rates. We also found that timely second-dose completion rates decreased over time. This may reflect differences between early adopters of vaccination and those who delayed vaccination, perhaps through vaccine hesitancy or other factors.

High rates of second-dose uptake among disadvantaged minoritized groups—especially Latinos, who received culturally and language-congruent support—highlight the important role of community-based vaccination initiatives. Although this initiative positively affected Latinos in the Baltimore area, the model of this intervention could be replicated to produce broader public health effects on a larger scale. Mobile and community-based models of care that meet patients at trusted sites can help promote health equity and could be adapted to provide other health services. AJPH

ABOUT THE AUTHORS

Cassandra Parent, Benjamin F. Bigelow, Stephen D. Sisson, and Kathleen R. Page are with the Johns Hopkins University School of Medicine, Baltimore, MD. Diego Martínez is with the School of Industrial Engineering, Pontificia Universidad Católica de Valparaíso, Chile. Cui Yang is with Rutgers University School of Public Health, Newark, NJ.

CORRESPONDENCE

Correspondence should be sent to Kathleen Page, MD, 600 N Wolfe St, Phipps 540, Baltimore, MD 21287 (e-mail: kpage2@jhmi.edu). Reprints can be ordered at http://www.ajph.org by clicking the "Reprints" link.

PUBLICATION INFORMATION

Full Citation: Parent C, Bigelow BF, Sisson SD, Martínez D, Yang C, Page KR. Timely second-dose completion of mRNA COVID-19 vaccination at community-based and mobile vaccine clinics in Maryland. *Am J Public Health*. 2023;113(9): 947–951.

Acceptance Date: May 11, 2023.

DOI: https://doi.org/10.2105/AJPH.2023.307338

CONTRIBUTORS

C. Parent performed study conceptualization and design, data analysis and interpretation, and manuscript writing. B. F. Bigelow preformed study design, data acquisition and interpretation, and manuscript revision. S. D. Sisson performed study design, data interpretation, and manuscript revision. D. Martínez and C. Yang performed study design, data analysis and interpretation, and manuscript revision. K. R. Page performed study conceptualization and design, data analysis and interpretation, and manuscript revision.

ACKNOWLEDGMENTS

Research reported in this article was supported by the National Institutes of Health (NIH awards U01MD017412, R01MD017364, and K24NR020508).

We acknowledge the many volunteers and the COVID-19 mobile vaccination team: Alejandra Flores-Miller, Ana Ortega Meza, Melissa Cuesta, Mervin Ruiz, MC Fortunato, Matt Franco. We are grateful to Bishop Bruce Lewandowski and Father Walker Ako for providing us space at the Sacred Heart Church and to the community members who participated in this work. This work would not have been possible without advocacy and support from the Esperanza Center, the Mayor's Office of Immigrant Affairs, the Maryland Department of Health, and Baltimore Latinos Unidos.

Note. The findings and conclusions in this article are those of the authors and do not necessarily represent the official position of the NIH.

CONFLICTS OF INTEREST

The authors have no conflicts of interest to report.

HUMAN PARTICIPANT PROTECTION

This study was reviewed and approved by the Johns Hopkins School of Medicine institutional review board (IRB00318866).

REFERENCES

1. Hill L, Artiga S. COVID-19 cases and deaths by race/ethnicity: current data and changes over time. Kaiser Family Foundation. August 22, 2022. Available at: https://www.kff.org/coronavirus-covid-19/issue-brief/covid-19-cases-and-deaths-by-race-ethnicity-current-data-and-changes-over-time. Accessed December 18, 2022.
2. Ross J, Diaz CM, Starrels JL. The disproportionate burden of COVID-19 for immigrants in the Bronx, New York. *JAMA Intern Med*. 2020;180(8):1043–1044. https://doi.org/10.1001/jamainternmed.2020.2131
3. Hamel L, Artiga S, Safarpour A, et al. KFF COVID-19 Vaccine Monitor: COVID-19 vaccine access, information, and experiences among Hispanic adults in the US. Kaiser Family Foundation. May 12, 2021. Available at: https://www.kff.org/coronavirus-covid-19/poll-finding/kff-covid-19-vaccine-monitor-access-information-experiences-hispanic-adults. Accessed December 18, 2022.
4. Bigelow BF, Martínez DA, Phillips K, et al. Coalition of faith leaders, community organizations, and governmental organizations to implement a COVID-19 campaign in a Latino neighborhood, Baltimore, Maryland, 2020–2021. *Am J Public Health*. 2022;112(suppl 9):S913–S917. https://doi.org/10.2105/AJPH.2022.307074

5. Bigelow BF, Saxton RE, Martínez DA, et al. High uptake and series completion of COVID-19 vaccine at community-based vaccination for Latinos with limited English proficiency. *J Public Health Manag Pract.* 2022;28(6):E789–E794. https://doi.org/10.1097/PHH.0000000000001625
6. Lester RT, Ritvo P, Mills EJ, et al. Effects of a mobile phone short message service on antiretroviral treatment adherence in Kenya (WelTel Kenya1): a randomised trial. *Lancet.* 2010;376(9755):1838–1845. https://doi.org/10.1016/S0140-6736(10)61997-6
7. *CBS.* Maryland institutes stricter vaccine protocols for workers at hospitals, nursing homes. August 18, 2021. Available at: https://www.cbsnews.com/baltimore/news/maryland-institutes-stricter-vaccine-protocols-at-hospitals-nursing-homes. Accessed May 27, 2023.
8. Ndugga N, Hill L, Artiga S, et al. Latest data on COVID-19 vaccinations by race/ethnicity. Kaiser Family Foundation. July 14, 2022. Available at: https://www.kff.org/coronavirus-covid-19/issue-brief/latest-data-on-covid-19-vaccinations-by-race-ethnicity. Accessed December 18, 2022.
9. Bradley T, Grundberg E, Selvarangan R, et al. Antibody responses after a single dose of SARS-CoV-2 mRNA vaccine. *N Engl J Med.* 2021;384(20):1959–1961. https://doi.org/10.1056/NEJMc2102051
10. Meng L, Murthy NC, Murthy BP, et al. Factors associated with delayed or missed second-dose mRNA COVID-19 vaccination among persons ≥12 years of age, United States. *Emerg Infect Dis.* 2022;28(8):1633–1641. https://doi.org/10.3201/eid2808.220557

An Alarming Trend in US Population Health

Kenneth Rochel de Camargo, MD, PhD

ABOUT THE AUTHOR

Kenneth Rochel de Camargo is a professor with the Instituto de Medicina Social, Universidade do Estado do Rio de Janeiro, Rio de Janeiro, Brazil, and is an AJPH *associate editor.*

See also US Life Expectancy, pp. 952–980.

This special section was motivated by Woolf's (p. 970 in this issue of *AJPH*) analysis of the widening gap in life expectancy between the United States and many other countries. The relatively poor performance of the United States in terms of certain population health indicators (e.g., life expectancy) is widely acknowledged, as Woolf himself registers, to the point of figuring in popular television series, as Remington (p. 956) reminds us. Woolf's work, however, adds to the extant arguments a widened analysis that extends further in time and geography, including comparisons to countries not usually contemplated in such analyses and bringing in-country comparisons as well. He shows that the relatively poor performance of the United States in this area began earlier than previously thought and is getting worse, that the disadvantages are not just in comparison with richer countries, and that although two regions of the United States (i.e., South and Midwest) are the major contributors to this state of affairs, all of the nine regions of the country are outperformed by other nations.

The editorials presented in this issue further extend and enhance Woolf's call for a debate. I present some of the more salient points of the editorials and emphasize the political message implicit in the discussion.

Some of the authors take a critical approach, for instance, focusing on the use of life expectancy in the comparisons. Case (p. 964) makes the most stringent critique, reminding us that this indicator is highly sensitive to modifications in early life mortality and that the available data might be faulty, given differences in mortality registry systems in the various countries used in the comparisons. However, Case does acknowledge that life expectancy is a useful, albeit "blunt," tool for such comparisons, and Aburto and Vigezzi (p. 967) add that it is an indicator that allows reliable comparisons over time and different populations. Aburto and Vigezzi also stress that Woolf's analyses did not look into differences by sex and age groups.

With regard specifically to the impact of infant mortality on life expectancy, two of the cited countries that made major progress in the period studied by Woolf—Uruguay and South Korea—have surpassed the United States in recent years: according to the United Nations Interagency Group for Child Mortality Estimation, the estimates for this indicator in 2021 were for Uruguay, South Korea, and the United States, respectively, 4.99, 2.47, and 5.36 per 1000 births (https://childmortality.org). It thus follows that Farina (p. 954) is correct in his assessment that at least part of the gains in life expectancy of the first two countries are attributable to progress in areas such as vaccination and sanitation, but the United States currently lags behind in this aspect as well.

Gaydosh (p. 959) highlights the fact that midlife (aged 25–64 years) deaths are a major contribution to the relatively poor performance of the United States in terms of life expectancy. As she states, this is a period that we expect to be characterized by a low risk of death, and yet deaths in this age bracket from many preventable causes have a major impact on overall mortality in the country.

Shanahan and Copeland (p. 961) call attention to the pitfalls of making such wide-ranging comparisons but acknowledge the value of Woolf's work, commenting that when the many relatively poor US socioeconomic indicators are considered, one wonders how the country does not fare even worse in terms of life expectancy. Both Gaydosh and Case highlight gaps in educational status, which are correlated with a starker gradient in health and mortality. This correlation might arise from a confounding with socioeconomic status, or it could be a direct contribution to poor quality of life, which in turn would be a determinant of the so-called deaths of despair.

The in-country comparisons Woolf makes were stressed in practically all of the editorials, especially for looking in more detail at which policies and conditions might explain this sorry state of affairs. The editorials also acknowledge the role of socioeconomic issues—in particular the widening economic inequality in the US population and the

AJPH September 2023, Vol 113, No. 9

erosion of welfare policies—as distal causes of the overall deterioration of the health status of a large part of the country's population as reflected by the lack of progress in life expectancy.

And here perhaps lie the greatest strength and contribution of Woolf's work and the accompanying editorials: as they shed light on a specific public health issue, they constitute a call to action as well. Shanahan and Copeland mention the contrast between European social democracies and US neoliberal economic policies, hinting at what could be done to reduce the observed gap—although it should be noted that in the past four decades even in those countries the neoliberal juggernaut has made inroads as well, bringing back social problems that seemed to have been solved.

Nevertheless, Remington poignantly asks who cares. Public health will do its share; it will point out where the problems are and help to mitigate some of the consequences, but the root causes of widening socioeconomic inequality and the problems it brings about are political and economic in nature and need to be tackled at those levels. In Remington's words, "Woolf's research may galvanize these people [i.e., those who do care] to work even harder" (p. 957). AJPH

CORRESPONDENCE

Correspondence should be sent to Kenneth Rochel de Camargo, Professor, Universidade do Estado do Rio de Janeiro, Instituto de Medicina Social, CEP 20550-013 Rua São Francisco Xavier, 524 / 7° andar / Bloco D—Maracanã, Rio de Janeiro, RJ 25.559-900 Brazil (e-mail: kenneth@uerj.br; kencamargo@gmail.com). Reprints can be ordered at http://www.ajph.org by clicking the "Reprints" link.

PUBLICATION INFORMATION

Full Citation: Rochel de Camargo K. An alarming trend in US population health. *Am J Public Health*. 2023;113(9):952–953.

Acceptance Date: June 26, 2023.

DOI: https://doi.org/10.2105/AJPH.2023.307378

ACKNOWLEDGMENTS

The author's research is funded by the Conselho Nacional de Desenvolvimento Científico e Tecnológico and the Universidade do Estado do Rio de Janeiro.

CONFLICTS OF INTEREST

The author has no conflicts of interest to declare.

Trends in Life Expectancy: Learning From International Comparisons

Mateo P. Farina, PhD

ABOUT THE AUTHOR

Mateo P. Farina is with the School of Gerontology, University of Southern California, Los Angeles, and with the Department of Human Development and Family Sciences, University of Texas at Austin.

See also US Life Expectancy, pp. 952–980.

In recent years, health scholars have raised the alarm about the worsening of population health in the United States as shown by the stagnation and recent decline in US life expectancy, which began in the 1990s. To illustrate the poor performance of the United States, scholars have compared changes in US life expectancy to those of other countries with similar levels of economic development, but this approach has some limitations. Woolf (p. 970 in this issue of *AJPH*) takes a more expansive perspective to address some of these limitations by (1) comparing the United States to countries with a broader array of social, economic, and political contexts, and (2) showing changes across specific periods of time from 1933 to 2021. This study adds rich descriptive information to situate US health within a broader global context, and it shows the underlying dynamic nature of changes in life expectancy over the last 88 years.

Comparisons of life expectancy between the United States and other countries have many challenges, especially when interpretation is considered. Prior scholars have compared the United States to a more limited set of countries with similar social and economic development—including many European countries, Canada, Australia, and Japan—to highlight stark differences between the stagnation and worsening of health in the United States since the 1970s and continued improvement in other countries with similar levels of resources.[1,2] This approach provides the background for continued scientific speculation as to why the United States continues to lag other "peer countries." The worsening of US population health has in part been attributed to disinvestments in the population, with less generous social welfare programs beginning in the 1970s.[3]

However, Woolf's study extends this perspective to show that declines in US health are not limited to social and political changes that started in the 1970s, but rather originate in the preceding decades. This point is exemplified by the lower gains in life expectancy compared with those of other countries even during the periods of improvement. Thus, it provides the basis for a broader discussion around the slowing of life expectancy gains prior to stagnation and decline in recent decades. For example, why did the significant social and health policy investments made from the New Deal in the 1930s to the Great Society of the 1960s not produce levels of improvement in the United States similar to those of other countries? Additionally, had entitlement programs such as Social Security and Medicaid never been passed, would US life expectancy appear even worse today? This perspective provides the basis for further exploration of the impact of health and social policies on population health, while providing a renewed critique of a period often characterized by more generous social investment.

Additionally, this study also provides the basis for evaluating changes within a broader global context. For example, life expectancy in South Korea increased from 52.4 years in 1950 to 78.5 years in 2005, transforming the country from a place with low performance to one of the highest-performing places in a matter of some 50 years,[4] eventually surpassing the United States. This leads to further questions about why life expectancy gains were rapid in other areas of the world or, relatedly, more modest in the United States. To better understand these phenomena, scholars might compare changes in age-specific mortality rates and their contributions to overall health metrics. The rapid improvements in life expectancy in countries like South Korea and Uruguay may be driven by significant improvements in infant and childhood mortality. If this is the case, then the rapid increases for other countries could also be interpreted as a major public health success that resulted from vaccination campaigns and sanitation improvements. Under this scenario, the public health improvements that rapidly increased life expectancy in other countries had already been implemented in the United States—other countries were simply catching up.[5]

Concomitantly, whether the United States continues to lag behind other countries because of higher maternal mortality rates[6] and greater exposures to violence, accidents, and alcohol[7,8] from young adulthood to midlife may provide additional insight into which policies may improve population health metrics. Thus, although life expectancy matters and provides an important health metric to allow for comparisons across countries, changes in mortality across age distributions would provide additional insight. This examination would be similar to prior studies that have used comparable approaches to better understand changes in educational inequalities in life expectancy in the United States.[9]

Lastly, Woolf's study highlights the uniqueness of the US political and social context. Changes in US life expectancy could be observed at the regional and state level, with the poorest performance among South-Central and Midwest regions. Importantly, he also shows that although states have stark differences in life expectancy, with some being equivalent to Austria and others to Mauritius, no state performed better in recent years than it had in previous years, and all contributed to the relative decline in US life expectancy ranking compared with other countries. This observation shifts the conversation around states with "poor" and "good" performance, and instead emphasizes the point that even states with "good" performance have contributed to the decline in US life expectancy ranking. It brings back the question of policies. What additional state policies might further contribute to improvements, even among better-performing states? Additionally, are further changes even possible given the limited ability of states to raise and spend money to pass and fund social welfare programs, or the seemingly growing political impasse at the federal level?

Altogether, Woolf's study expands the conversation on the poor performance of the United States in terms of life expectancy, and shows how this process may be dynamic, pointing to both historical changes and differences across country contexts. By providing rich descriptive information on changes in life expectancy in the United States and other countries, it spurs more questions that may lead to thinking about how to improve population health in the United States and what lessons can be learned by evaluating changes in health metrics across a variety of contexts. AJPH

CORRESPONDENCE

Correspondence should be sent to Mateo P. Farina, 108 E Dean Keeton St, Austin, TX 78712 (e-mail: mateo.farina@austin.utexas.edu). Reprints can be ordered at http://www.ajph.org by clicking the "Reprints" link.

PUBLICATION INFORMATION

Full Citation: Farina MP. Trends in life expectancy: learning from international comparisons. *Am J Public Health*. 2023;113(9):954–955.

Acceptance Date: June 13, 2023.

DOI: https://doi.org/10.2105/AJPH.2023.307365

ACKNOWLEDGMENTS

This work was supported by the National Institute of Aging (K99AG076964).

CONFLICTS OF INTEREST

The author has no conflicts of interest to report.

REFERENCES

1. Woolf SH, Aron L. Failing health of the United States. *BMJ*. 2018;360:k496. https://doi.org/10.1136/bmj.k496
2. Ho JY, Hendi AS. Recent trends in life expectancy across high income countries: retrospective observational study [erratum in *BMJ*. 2018;362:k3622]. *BMJ*. 2018;362:k2562. https://doi.org/10.1136/bmj.k2562
3. Montez JK, Beckfield J, Cooney JK, et al. US state policies, politics, and life expectancy. *Milbank Q*. 2020;98(3):668–699. https://doi.org/10.1111/1468-0009.12469
4. Yang S, Khang YH, Harper S, Davey Smith G, Leon DA, Lynch J. Understanding the rapid increase in life expectancy in South Korea. *Am J Public Health*. 2010;100(5):896–903. https://doi.org/10.2105/AJPH.2009.160341
5. Bhatia A, Krieger N, Subramanian SV. Learning from history about reducing infant mortality: contrasting the centrality of structural interventions to early 20th-century successes in the United States to their neglect in current global initiatives. *Milbank Q*. 2019;97(1):285–345. https://doi.org/10.1111/1468-0009.12376
6. MacDorman MF, Declercq E, Cabral H, Morton C. Is the United States maternal mortality rate increasing? Disentangling trends from measurement issues. *Obstet Gynecol*. 2016;128(3):447–455. https://doi.org/10.1097/AOG.0000000000001556
7. Spillane S, Shiels MS, Best AF, et al. Trends in alcohol-induced deaths in the United States, 2000–2016. *JAMA Netw Open*. 2020;3(2):e1921451. https://doi.org/10.1001/jamanetworkopen.2019.21451
8. Grinshteyn E, Hemenway D. Violent death rates: the US compared with other high-income OECD countries, 2010. *Am J Med*. 2016;129(3):266–273. https://doi.org/10.1016/j.amjmed.2015.10.025
9. Brown DC, Hayward MD, Montez JK, Humme RA, Chiu CT, Hidajat MM. The significance of education for mortality compression in the United States. *Demography*. 2012;49(3):819–840. https://doi.org/10.1007/s13524-012-0104-1

Trends in US Life Expectancy: Falling Behind and Failing to Act

Patrick L. Remington, MD, MPH

ABOUT THE AUTHOR

Patrick L. Remington is with the Department of Population Health Sciences, School of Medicine and Public Health, University of Wisconsin, Madison.

See also US Life Expectancy, pp. 952–980.

"We have met the enemy and he is us."
—*Pogo (Pogo comic strip, April 22, 1970)*

The goal of public health is to ensure conditions that support long and healthy lives for all. Although no single measure can determine our progress toward achieving this goal, countries around the globe have used life expectancy as a summary measure of health, as it is the outcome of the multiple upstream determinants of health, including health behaviors, health care, social and economic factors, and the environment.[1,2]

The study by Woolf, "Falling Behind: The Growing Gap in Life Expectancy Between the United States and Other Countries, 1933–2021" appearing in this issue of *AJPH* (p. 970), is a comprehensive assessment of the trends in life expectancy in the United States compared with other countries. While reading this article, I was reminded of the scene in the HBO series *The Newsroom* from a decade ago[3] in which Will McAvoy (Jeff Daniels), anchor and managing editor of a news program, responded to a student who asked, "Can you say why America is the greatest country in the world?" He shocked the audience by saying, "It's not the greatest country in the world" and substantiating this claim by citing poor ranks in life expectancy and other measures of population health.

THE TRENDS

Woolf's study adds to a growing literature that shows that US life expectancy has fallen behind that of many other countries. Woolf contrasted life expectancy trends in the United States with trends in 236 other countries. The good news is that from 1974 to 2019, US life expectancy increased from 72 to 79 years; the bad news is that our rank dropped from 15th to 40th during this time. In fact, since 1930, 56 countries on six continents surpassed the United States in life expectancy.

Woolf also shows where these problems are the greatest, suggesting that the US life expectancy disadvantage is owing primarily to conditions in the Midwest and the South Central states. Although this is true, it paints the problem with too broad a brush, as there is significant variability in these regions, states, and even counties, both in present rates and in long-term trends.

Data supporting this are now easily accessible in the Centers for Disease Control and Prevention's National Center for Health Statistics data visualization gallery, which clearly demonstrates which communities have the lowest life expectancies.[4] For example, of 1409 census tracts in Wisconsin, the tracts with the highest and lowest life expectancies are both in Milwaukee County (89.0 years in tract 703 in Whitefish Bay vs 65.9 years in tract 1705 in South Milwaukee; Figure 1). Leaders in every community across this country should use the data visualization gallery to identify the areas in greatest need and address their needs.

IMPLICATIONS OF THIS RESEARCH

In his discussion, Woolf cites the 2013 National Research Council report[5] that describes five domains that might explain the US health disadvantage: health systems, individual behaviors, socioeconomic factors, the environment, and policies and social values. It is unlikely that only one of these factors accounts for our disadvantage in life expectancy; rather, it results from disadvantages in all these domains.

Woolf aptly points out that these factors are outcomes of US policies that began in the 1970s with the intention of promoting entrepreneurial freedom and deregulation, redistributing wealth from the middle to the upper class, and curbing government's ability to broaden access to education, health care, and human services.[6] We need look no further than our nation's response to the COVID-19 pandemic, which exposed long-standing problems with the US health care system, including barriers to accessing care, uncontrolled costs, unacceptable quality, widespread disparities and inequities, and the marginalization of public health.[7,8]

If there is a criticism of Woolf's article, it is the author's reluctance to make

AJPH September 2023, Vol 113, No. 9

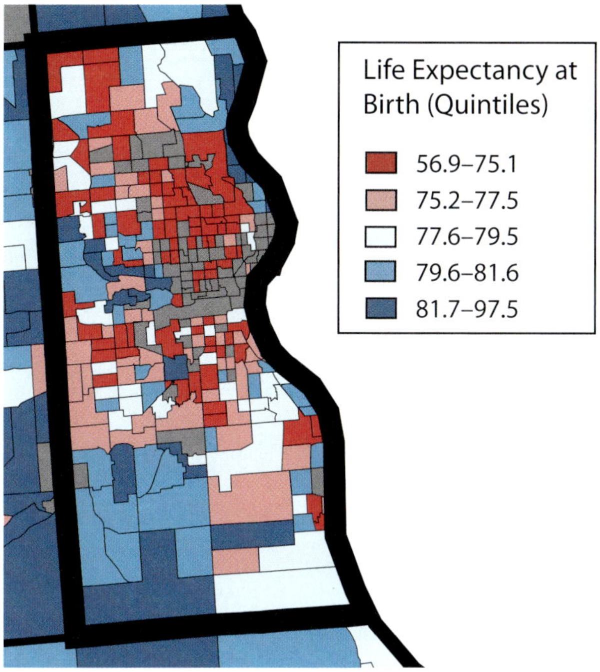

FIGURE 1— **Life Expectancy at Birth, by Census Tract: Milwaukee County, WI, 2010–2015**

Source. Centers for Disease Control and Prevention.[4]

causal inferences about these factors. Although researchers must be free from bias, the core of any policy change is a strong understanding of the epidemiologic data and a critical evaluation of the data's strengths and weaknesses.[9] We will never know for certain what causes the drop in US life expectancy ranking, as there are too many variables and potentially confounding factors to consider, but we cannot continue on the same course and expect different outcomes.

Woolf states, "A prudent first step [toward improving US life expectancy] would be to examine policies that have enabled other countries to consistently outperform the United States for decades" (p. 979). I would go further and recommend that we change course as a nation now and adopt the policies that have been shown to be effective in other countries for achieving longer and healthier lives for all: robust investments in public education, well-funded social service programs, universal health care, and safety net programs for those who fall through the cracks.

OUR FAILURE TO ACT

There is compelling evidence that we will not achieve our public health goals without a major change in our social, economic, and political systems. However, there are some who openly state that they do not share these goals. Instead, they subscribe to a market justice philosophy that holds that there are simply winners and losers and that it is not the responsibility of governments to intervene. They shun collective action, perhaps because this would require them to contribute more to the solutions than those in need. Woolf's findings may be of little interest to these people because they affect others and not them.

There are also those who care deeply and have dedicated their lives to making our country better for all. They subscribe to a social justice approach that holds that all people deserve to have their basic human needs of food, shelter, and health care met. They support collective action, including policies that ensure access to these basic human needs. They demonstrate this philosophy by supporting public education and policies that may not be in their self-interest but are intended to benefit others. Woolf's research may galvanize these people to work even harder.

There are, furthermore, those who say that they care and support progressive causes but do not translate this philosophy into action. They, perhaps, have a great job and choose to live in a segregated, affluent, and safe neighborhood. They may send their children to private schools and hire financial advisers who work to preserve their wealth through tax avoidance strategies. They may express concern about those who are struggling to make ends meet, but their actions focus on self-interest and preserving the status quo. This failure to act helps fuel inequality in the United States[10] and is perhaps the single most important obstacle preventing this nation from changing course and reversing the trends toward shorter lives and poorer health for those who can least afford it. AJPH

CORRESPONDENCE

Correspondence should be sent to Patrick L. Remington, MD, MPH, 610 Walnut St, Rm 1007, Department of Population Health Sciences, School of Medicine and Public Health, University of Wisconsin, Madison, WI 53726 (e-mail: plreming@wisc.edu). Reprints can be ordered at http://www.ajph.org by clicking the "Reprints" link.

PUBLICATION INFORMATION

Full Citation: Remington PL. Trends in US life expectancy: falling behind and failing to act. *Am J Public Health.* 2023;113(9):956–958.

Acceptance Date: June 13, 2023.

DOI: https://doi.org/10.2105/AJPH.2023.307366

ACKNOWLEDGMENTS

P. L. Remington is supported by the Department of Population Health Sciences, School of Medicine and Public Health, University of Wisconsin, Madison.

CONFLICTS OF INTEREST

The author has no conflicts of interest to declare.

REFERENCES

1. Parrish RG. Measuring population health outcomes. *Prev Chronic Dis.* 2010;7(4):A71.
2. Remington PL, Catlin BB, Gennuso KP. The county health rankings: rationale and methods. *Popul Health Metr.* 2015;13:11. https://doi.org/10.1186/s12963-015-0044-2
3. Sorkin A, creator. *The Newsroom.* HBO. June 24, 2012.
4. Centers for Disease Control and Prevention. Life expectancy at birth for US states and census tracts, 2010–2015. Available at: https://www.cdc.gov/nchs/data-visualization/life-expectancy. Accessed June 8, 2023.
5. Woolf SH, Aron L, eds. *US Health in International Perspective: Shorter Lives, Poorer Health.* Washington, DC: National Academies Press; 2013.
6. Williams C, Maruthappu M. "Healthconomic crises": public health and neoliberal economic crises. *Am J Public Health.* 2013;103(1):7–9. https://doi.org/10.2105/AJPH.2012.300956
7. Geyman J. COVID-19 has revealed America's broken health care system: what can we learn? *Int J Health Serv.* 2021;51(2):188–194. https://doi.org/10.1177/0020731420985640
8. Navarro V. The consequences of neoliberalism in the current pandemic. *Int J Health Serv.* 2020; 50(3):271–275. https://doi.org/10.1177/0020731420925449
9. Davis FG, Peterson CE, Bandiera F, Carter-Pokras O, Brownson RC. How do we more effectively move epidemiology into policy action? *Ann Epidemiol.* 2012;22(6):413–416. https://doi.org/10.1016/j.annepidem.2012.04.004
10. Liberal hypocrisy is fueling American inequality. Here's how. NYT Opinion. November 9, 2021. Available at: https://www.youtube.com/watch?v=hNDgcjVGHIw. Accessed June 8, 2023.

Failing Population Health: US Life Expectancy Falling Behind

Lauren Gaydosh, PhD

ABOUT THE AUTHOR

Lauren Gaydosh is an assistant professor in the Department of Sociology, faculty scholar at the Population Research Center, and affiliate at the Center on Aging and Population Sciences at The University of Texas at Austin.

See also US Life Expectancy, pp. 952–980.

Health in the United States is failing by most metrics that demographers use to monitor the well-being of populations. In 2020, life expectancy at birth declined to a level last observed nearly two decades earlier.[1] Infant mortality ranks worst among peer countries, and maternal mortality is triple the Organisation for Economic Co-operation and Development (OECD) average.[2] Mortality among individuals in midlife has been increasing, for several decades among some groups.[3] Americans not only live shorter lives, but our lives are also less healthy on average, with rising rates of diabetes, hypertension, obesity, and mental health conditions.[2] While troubling in their own right, these trends also diverge from most of the global community, which has seen continual improvements in population health. As Woolf describes in this issue of *AJPH* (p. 970), the United States continues to fall behind other countries, moving from 12th to 46th in terms of rank over the period from 1950 to the present.

US HEALTH POOR AND UNEQUAL

The ranking and trends in US life expectancy belie important heterogeneity that clarify US population health not just as poor and declining but also as characterized by stark inequalities.[4] Indeed, Woolf highlights the role of geography, replicating the well-established disadvantage of states in the US South and Midwest. Additional differentiation by age, race/ethnicity, and socioeconomic status further demonstrates the current state of US population health as determined by social and structural factors that disproportionately shorten the lives of our country's marginalized populations.

The overall trend of deteriorating population health in the United States is particularly worrisome when we understand that rising midlife mortality is responsible for declines in life expectancy and causing the United States to fall behind other countries.[5] The midlife period (ages 25–64 years) should be characterized by relatively good health and low risk of death, with chronic conditions typically accumulating toward the end of this life stage and death forestalled until old age. Yet, midlife health in the United States is facing a uniquely disturbing crisis, with individuals dying well before old age and of causes that are largely preventable, such as suicide, chronic liver disease, and accidental poisoning.[3] The fact that these causes of death are avoidable points to systemic failures that exclude individuals from successful social integration and cause individuals to detach from social institutions.[6]

In addition to the role of preventable causes of death, part of what made rising midlife mortality so striking was that it was observed among a population that is typically advantaged in the United States—non-Hispanic White adults.[7] This fact, coupled with the narrowing of the Black–White mortality gap over the last several decades, may have given the false impression that racial and ethnic health disparities were no longer cause for concern. Yet, Black and Hispanic individuals experienced similar if not higher rates and trajectories of substance use behaviors and mental health problems across adolescence, early adulthood, and as they entered midlife.[8,9] Moreover, starting about a decade ago, midlife mortality also began to rise among minoritized racial and ethnic groups, oftentimes outpacing increases among non-Hispanic White adults.[10] Finally, the disproportionate burden and impact of the COVID-19 pandemic erased nearly all of the previous progress in reducing racial/ethnic health disparities.[11]

Even as overall US life expectancy declined, individuals with high socioeconomic status, measured in terms of education, income, or occupation, continued to extend their longevity.[3] The result is a steepening of the socioeconomic gradient in health and mortality, with the differences between the advantaged and disadvantaged now even more pronounced. As Woolf mentions, this mirrors other social and economic trends of increasing inequality.

PERSISTENT AND GROWING EDUCATIONAL DISPARITIES

Educational attainment specifically plays an increasingly important role,[4]

AJPH September 2023, Vol 113, No. 9

the effects of which can be observed across the life course. In a nationally representative and diverse sample of US individuals born 1974 to 1982, the National Longitudinal Study of Adolescent to Adult Health (Add Health), I measured six physical and mental health and health behavior outcomes. This cohort was initially interviewed in adolescence in 1994 (ages 13–20 years) and followed up over four additional collection waves, most recently in 2016 to 2018 (ages 33–43 years). I present in Figure A (available as a supplement to the online version of this article at https://ajph.org) the median level or prevalence of each condition at each age, separately for those with and without a college degree, using cubic splines to flexibly fit the age pattern. We see the divergence in health between those with and without a four-year college degree, starting early in the life course and persisting or widening as individuals age into midlife.

We also see evidence of an increasing burden of poor health as individuals age into midlife, consistent with the observed trends in midlife health and mortality.[3] With body mass index (BMI) and self-rated health in particular, we see worsening physical health as individuals age into midlife. After an initial peak in late adolescence, depressive symptoms follow a similar pattern, with increases across early and into mid-adulthood. Suicidal ideation, heavy drinking (more than the recommended daily limit on average), and any marijuana use in the last year all share a similar peak in adolescence or early adulthood, reaching relative stability across the late 20s and 30s. Even as the prevalence of health behaviors plateaus, the differentiation between educational groups remains or even widens.

As population health scholars and policymakers continue to work on documenting, understanding, and addressing declines in US life expectancy, future explanations and solutions must attend to the role of midlife health and the persistence and widening of health inequities by race, ethnicity, and socioeconomic position. Promising directions for future effort would interrogate how such inequalities contribute to the international and intranational patterns documented in Woolf's work. Such comparative work illuminates our current position as historically and politically situated and highlights the possibility and promise of alternative population health futures rather than failures. AJPH

CORRESPONDENCE

Correspondence should be sent to Lauren Gaydosh, 305 E 23rd St, Austin, TX 78712-1699 (e-mail: lauren.gaydosh@austin.utexas.edu). Reprints can be ordered at https://ajph.org by clicking the "Reprints" link.

PUBLICATION INFORMATION

Full Citation: Gaydosh L. Failing population health: US life expectancy falling behind. *Am J Public Health*. 2023;113(9):959–960.

Acceptance Date: June 20, 2023.

DOI: https://doi.org/10.2105/AJPH.2023.307370

ACKNOWLEDGMENTS

This research was supported by grant P30AG066614, awarded to the Center on Aging and Population Sciences at The University of Texas at Austin by the National Institute on Aging, and by grant P2CHD042849, awarded to the Population Research Center at The University of Texas at Austin by the Eunice Kennedy Shriver National Institute of Child Health and Human Development.

Note. The content is solely the responsibility of the authors and does not necessarily represent the official views of the National Institutes of Health.

CONFLICTS OF INTEREST

There are no conflicts of interest to report.

REFERENCES

1. Murphy SL, Kochanek KD, Xu J, Arias E. Mortality in the United States, 2020. 2021. Available at: https://www.cdc.gov/nchs/products/index.htm. Accessed June 11, 2023.
2. Gunja M, Gumas E, Williams R III. US health care from a global perspective, 2022: accelerating spending, worsening outcomes. Commonwealth Fund. 2023. Available at: https://www.commonwealthfund.org/publications/issue-briefs/2023/jan/us-health-care-global-perspective-2022. Accessed June 30, 2023.
3. National Academies of Sciences, Engineering, and Medicine. *High and Rising Mortality Rates Among Working-Age Adults.* Washington, DC: The National Academies Press; 2021. https://doi.org/10.17226/25976
4. Gutin I, Hummer RA. Social inequality and the future of US life expectancy. *Annu Rev Sociol.* 2021;47(1):501–520. https://doi.org/10.1146/annurev-soc-072320-100249
5. Avendano M, Kawachi I. Why do Americans have shorter life expectancy and worse health than do people in other high-income countries? *Annu Rev Public Health.* 2014;35(1):307–325. https://doi.org/10.1146/annurev-publhealth-032013-182411
6. Shanahan L, Hill SN, Gaydosh LM, et al. Does despair really kill? A roadmap for an evidence-based answer. *Am J Public Health.* 2019;109(6):854–858. https://doi.org/10.2105/AJPH.2019.305016
7. Case A, Deaton A. Rising morbidity and mortality in midlife among White non-Hispanic Americans in the 21st century. *Proc Natl Acad Sci U S A.* 2015;112(49):15078–15083. https://doi.org/10.1073/pnas.1518393112
8. Hargrove TW, Halpern CT, Gaydosh L, et al. Race/ethnicity, gender, and trajectories of depressive symptoms across early- and mid-life among the Add Health cohort. *J Racial Ethn Health Disparities.* 2020;7(4):619–629. https://doi.org/10.1007/s40615-019-00692-8
9. Gaydosh L, Hummer RA, Hargrove TW, et al. The depths of despair among US adults entering midlife. *Am J Public Health.* 2019;109(5):774–780. https://doi.org/10.2105/AJPH.2019.305002
10. Woolf SH, Chapman D, Buchanich J, Bobby K. Changes in midlife death rates across racial and ethnic groups in the United States: systematic analysis of vital statistics. *BMJ.* 2018;362:k3096. https://doi.org/10.1136/bmj.k3096
11. Aburto JM, Tilstra AM, Floridi G, Dowd JB. Significant impacts of the COVID-19 pandemic on race/ethnic differences in US mortality. *Proc Natl Acad Sci U S A.* 2022;119(35):e2205813119. https://doi.org/10.1073/pnas.2205813119

A Deadly Drop in Rankings: How the United States Was Left Behind in Global Life Expectancy Trends

Lilly Shanahan, PhD, and William E. Copeland, PhD

ABOUT THE AUTHORS

Lilly Shanahan is with the Department of Psychology and the Jacobs Center for Productive Youth Development at the University of Zurich in Zurich, Switzerland. William E. Copeland is with the Department of Psychiatry at the University of Vermont, Burlington.

See also US Life Expectancy, pp. 952–980.

It has been a decade since the US life expectancy slowdown caught researchers' and the public's attention.[1] Initially, some research suggested that these trends were relatively straightforward, circumscribed, and time-limited.[2] Since then, much empirical work has suggested the opposite.[3]

US LIFE EXPECTANCY IN GLOBAL–HISTORICAL CONTEXT

Woolf's new analysis (p. 970) contributes to this evidence by masterfully describing cross-national trends in life expectancy, disaggregated by time and contextualized with data from a total of 236 countries over eight decades, to highlight the relative standing of the United States. He swings the lens away from specific causes of death, including the so-called "deaths of despair"[4] (suicides, drug poisonings, alcoholic liver disease), to provide a broader perspective on life expectancy.

This historical analysis reveals that while US life expectancy generally rose until about 2013, its life expectancy disadvantage (i.e., shorter lifespan than comparison countries) has increased since the mid-1950s, with a brief interruption of this trend from 1974 to 1982. Furthermore, no single US state has hit the median yearly increase in life expectancy of other populous countries (1960–2019 aggregate estimate in Woolf's Table 1, p. 976–977).

The steep increase in the US life expectancy disadvantage since 2010 is striking and has been subject to much debate. According to Woolf's analysis, the US life expectancy rank in 1933 was eighth. From 1977 to 1980, the United States placed 14th (2.2 to 2.4 years behind lead countries Norway and Japan). Much ground has been lost since then, with the United States placing 40th in 2019 (6.1 years behind lead country Hong Kong) and 46th in 2020 (7.8 years behind lead country Hong Kong). Indeed, between 2010 and 2021, the life expectancy difference between the United States and the lead country increased by four years.

Woolf's paper also features noteworthy domestic analyses: the Midwest and South US Census regions (24 states) have been pronouncedly left behind. If Mississippi were considered a country, it would have placed 79th in the world in 2019. While all states have contributed to the growing life expectancy disadvantage, the South and Midwest are much worse off than the Northeast and the West, where New York and California were relatively positive standouts.

Why has the full extent of the US life expectancy disadvantage gone unnoticed? Woolf impressively identified, merged, and analyzed three different extant data sources over eight decades to (1) compare countries' growth trends (slopes) rather than annual or decadal snapshots, (2) zoom out in historical time as far as records allowed, and (3) extend the analysis to countries with weaker economies that are typically excluded from such comparisons.

While the analyses were expertly conducted, a few things should be considered. First, estimates from all countries may not be of equal quality. Second, data aggregation into six phases reduces information in particular ways. Third, data for the 179 countries that never outranked the United States were not shown, with many located in Africa, Asia, and South America.

Provocative descriptive findings inevitably elicit questions about additional data analyses. For example, what age brackets contribute to the US life expectancy disadvantage? In comparative analyses with peer countries, US working-age mortality increased the most, but Americans of all ages are more likely to die (except, until recently, older Americans).[3,5] Furthermore, subgroup analyses typically find that non-Hispanic Blacks and American Indians and Alaska Natives have gaping life expectancy disadvantages within the United States compared with Whites and Asians, for example.[3] How do such racial/ethnic disparities compare with disadvantaged minority groups in peer countries? This question could be difficult to answer because these countries often historically had less diverse populations and different migration and immigration histories.

WHY LIFE EXPECTANCY ELSEWHERE HAS INCREASED MORE

Comparative analysis raises questions about causes of between-countries differences. A National Academies of Sciences, Engineering, and Medicine report details why life expectancy for working-aged US residents may have stalled.[3] But why has life expectancy elsewhere increased more steeply? Woolf's findings suggest that several wealthy European (e.g., Scandinavian) and Anglo-Saxon nations consistently outperformed the United States in life expectancy. From the 1950s to the 1970s, many European countries affected by World War II surpassed the United States. Many of these countries adopted social market economies, combining free market capitalism with social welfare policies and select regulations (e.g., of the labor market) aimed at achieving some level of financial security for the entire population. This approach contrasts with less regulated and less welfare-oriented US (neoliberalist) economic policies.[6]

There is likely no unitary cause for 20 additional nations surpassing US life expectancy between 1980 and 2019, but high rates of US drug poisonings, suicides, alcoholic liver disease, and homicides, and stalling progress in cardiovascular health likely contributed.[3] Surpassing countries included those recovering from the 1990s' wars in the Balkans and strong Asian and oil-based Middle Eastern economies. Notably, nine small countries exceeded the population threshold of 500 000 and surpassed the United States in life expectancy since the mid-1960s (e.g., Kuwait, Luxembourg, Macao). Adding these countries to the analysis dropped the US rank by nine points.

There are other questions about between-countries differences: How are various national indicators of income, education, health, and health care, and within-country inequalities in these indicators, linked with differences in life expectancy?[7] How do labor market conditions, social welfare, and other regulations affect these differences?[5] With the exception of (absolute) income, the United States lags behind in the rankings on many indicators, including obesity, smoking, incarceration, childhood poverty, adolescent pregnancy, and infant and maternal mortality. In turn, it scores highly on indicators of inequalities such as the Gini coefficient of income inequality. It is perhaps surprising that the United States does not rank lower in life expectancy.

The important demographic groundwork by Woolf and other scholars also stimulated research on how between-states policies contribute to life expectancy.[8,9] Immense between-states heterogeneity lends itself to examining which state policies change life expectancy (e.g., policies regarding labor, tobacco and other substances, environment, immigration, civil rights, and gun control).[8,9] By some prepandemic estimates, altering state policies could change the overall US life expectancy by two years. Thus, changes in state-level policy, and perhaps reducing between-states variability by adopting effective health-promoting policies, could lessen US life expectancy disadvantage and disparities significantly.[8] However, as the COVID-19 pandemic illustrated, once effective policies are identified, significant challenges remain regarding how to make these guidelines and regulations accessible to larger segments of the population and how to increase public buy-in.

MANY DIVERSE FACTORS INFLUENCE LIFE EXPECTANCY

Indeed, the COVID-19 pandemic exemplified that many factors, at multiple levels, combine to determine life-and-death questions.[10] These factors included preexisting conditions (e.g., extant policies and public health infrastructures, health vulnerabilities including obesity and poverty), newly implemented policies (e.g., social distancing), and individual behavior (e.g., vaccination uptake, policy adherence). Similarly, the US life expectancy disadvantage is attributable to multilevel, multifactorial causation,[3] which increases the challenges of identifying all of its drivers. However, this causal web also explains why the life expectancy disadvantage has been robust for decades and is exacerbated in the context of new risks (e.g., opioids, COVID-19 pandemic) and perhaps even self-perpetuates.[3] Indeed, premature deaths devastate families and communities, likely causing new trauma, which poses new health risks.[11]

Identifying and changing single (state) policies or psychological factors will likely be insufficient for reversing the US life expectancy disadvantage. Woolf's analysis suggests that understanding US population-level trends and their causes in a global–historical context could lead to a deeper appreciation of what is needed to change the US life expectancy disadvantage. AJPH

CORRESPONDENCE

Correspondence should be sent to Lilly Shanahan, Associate Professor, University of Zurich, Jacobs Center for Productive Youth Development, Andreasstrasse 15, PO Box 12, CH-8050 Zurich, Switzerland (e-mail: lilly.shanahan@uzh.ch). Reprints can be ordered at https://ajph.org by clicking the "Reprints" link.

PUBLICATION INFORMATION

Full Citation: Shanahan L, Copeland WE. A deadly drop in rankings: how the United States was left behind in global life expectancy trends. *Am J Public Health*. 2023;113(9):961–963.

Acceptance Date: June 13, 2023.

DOI: https://doi.org/10.2105/AJPH.2023.307367

CONTRIBUTORS

The authors contributed equally to this editorial.

ACKNOWLEDGMENTS

This work was supported by the National Institute of Mental Health (MH117559) and the National Institute on Drug Abuse (DA036523).

CONFLICTS OF INTEREST

The authors have no financial disclosures to report.

REFERENCES

1. National Research Council, Institute of Medicine, Woolf SH, Aaron L, eds. *US Health in International Perspective: Shorter Lives, Poorer Health*. Washington, DC: The National Academies Press; 2013.
2. Case A, Deaton A. Rising morbidity and mortality in midlife among White non-Hispanic Americans in the 21st century. *Proc Natl Acad Sci USA*. 2015; 112(49):15078–15083. https://doi.org/10.1073/pnas.1518393112
3. National Academies of Sciences, Engineering, and Medicine; Division of Behavioral and Social Sciences and Education; Committee on National Statistics; Committee on Population; Committee on Rising Midlife Mortality Rates and Socioeconomic Disparities; Becker T, Majmundar MK, Harris KM, eds. *High and Rising Mortality Rates Among Working-Age Adults*. Washington, DC: National Academies Press; 2021.
4. Case A, Deaton A. *Deaths of Despair and the Future of Capitalism*. Princeton, NJ: Princeton University Press; 2020.
5. Sterling P, Platt ML. Why deaths of despair are increasing in the US and not other industrial nations—insights from neuroscience and anthropology. *JAMA Psychiatry*. 2022;79(4):368–374. https://doi.org/10.1001/jamapsychiatry.2021.4209
6. Freeman T, Gesesew HA, Bambra C, et al. Why do some countries do better or worse in life expectancy relative to income? An analysis of Brazil, Ethiopia, and the United States of America. *Int J Equity Health*. 2020;19(1):202. https://doi.org/10.1186/s12939-020-01315-z
7. Chetty R, Stepner M, Abraham S, et al. The association between income and life expectancy in the United States, 2001–2014. *JAMA*. 2016;315(16): 1750–1766. https://doi.org/10.1001/jama.2016.4226
8. Montez JK, Beckfield J, Cooney JK, et al. US state policies, politics, and life expectancy. *Milbank Q*. 2020;98(3):668–699. https://doi.org/10.1111/1468-0009.12469
9. Woolf SH. The growing influence of state governments on population health in the United States. *JAMA*. 2022;327(14):1331–1332. https://doi.org/10.1001/jama.2022.3785
10. Schöley J, Aburto JM, Kashnitsky I, et al. Life expectancy changes since COVID-19. *Nat Hum Behav*. 2022;6(12):1649–1659. https://doi.org/10.1038/s41562-022-01450-3
11. Copeland WE, Shanahan L, Hinesley J, Aberg KA, Van Den Oord EJ, Costello EJ. Association of childhood trauma exposure with adult psychiatric disorders and functional outcomes. *JAMA Network Open*. 2018;1(7):e184493. https://doi.org/10.1001/jamanetworkopen.2018.4493

Something Related to Education May Hold the Key to Understanding What Is Ailing the United States

Anne Case, PhD, MPA

ABOUT THE AUTHOR

Anne Case is the Alexander Stewart 1886 Professor of Economics and Public Affairs, Emeritus, Princeton University, Princeton, NJ.

See also US Life Expectancy, pp. 952–980.

AJPH September 2023, Vol 113, No. 9

Woolf, in this issue of *AJPH* (p. 970), has done a great service in bringing additional attention to the poor state of American health, identifying periods of progress and stagnation in US life expectancy over the past 70 years and comparing outcomes in the United States with a large set of countries, one that includes not only the wealthy countries of Europe and the English-speaking world but also lower-income and non-Western countries. My comments on this work fall into two categories. First, discussing methodology and data, I provide some caveats on the comparisons presented. The term "data" should be reserved for information collected (not generated or modeled). The distinction is of first-order importance for policy. Second, I fill in additional details on US mortality, what we know about what is killing us, and where new research is leading. Life expectancy does not speak to cause of death, to who is dying, or to the underlying mechanisms, all information that is essential if we are to design good policies.

Woolf references many research studies that have focused on the gap in life expectancy between the United States and other rich countries over the past 30 or 40 years. He goes on to comment that research to date has made two implicit assumptions: (1) that only high-income countries have outperformed the United States in life expectancy, and (2) that the US disadvantage only dates to the 1980s or 1990s. I found this comment puzzling, given that there is a large literature on changes in life expectancy across both poor and rich countries, including the United States, using historical and contemporary data, where neither assumption comes into play (see Deaton and references there[1]).

One limit to comparisons between richer and poorer countries is a lack of civil registration and vital statistics systems in the latter. In 2014, the World Health Organization estimated that two thirds of all annual deaths (38 million of 56 million globally) were not registered, missing almost 50% of child deaths.[2] The Global Burden of Disease 2016 study evaluated the quality of mortality data from 1980 to 2016 and gave its highest quality ranking to only 25 of 195 countries queried—which limits the data available for informative analyses of this period.[3] Progress is being made in developing and upgrading civil registration and vital statistics systems globally, but it will take time before these systems have the wherewithal to provide data for close analysis.[4]

Where data are not collected, or are only partially or sporadically collected, many research teams have taken it upon themselves to estimate what might have been. There is a long and distinguished history of demography on how to do this, dating back to Coale and Demeny's model life tables[5] and, later, to limited parameter models of mortality by age. Despite the increasing sophistication, and the work done by Murray et al. at the Institute for Health Metrics and Evaluation (https://www.healthdata.org), there is a world of difference between using actual data from civil registration and vital statistics systems and numbers that are ultimately invented. For formulating policies, estimates of life expectancy generated by algorithm are unlikely to be adequate if only because, in many cases, the estimates are unresponsive to policy. Without data, it is not possible to evaluate the impact of health policies; mortality responses to policy changes will often not show up in modeled estimates.

Moreover, comparisons across countries with very different age, education, income, and burden of disease structures are less likely to be useful for policy purposes than comparisons between similar countries.

Woolf notes:

> Clarifying the timing and geographic scale of the US life expectancy disadvantage is important groundwork for investigating potential causes. For example, knowing the years when

> changes occurred in the slope—the rate of change in US life expectancy—is a prerequisite for future studies of period and cohort effects. (p. 971)

Perhaps. Life expectancy, aggregating mortality over all causes and ages into one index number, is useful as a broad gauge on how we are doing. But it is a blunt tool. Saving the life of an infant has a much larger effect on life expectancy than does saving a life at 30 years. Of course, Woolf is not making an ethical case for the use of life expectancy but a pragmatic case—that it can reveal something about the state of our health. But this feature of life expectancy, down-weighting mortality at higher ages, is especially important when comparing progress made by a poor country (which can bring life expectancy up relatively rapidly by reducing infant mortality) and progress made by a wealthy country (that has already reduced infant mortality and is working to reduce death from the chronic diseases that plague people at higher ages). The 20th century saw gains, plateaus, and losses in life expectancy owing to factors that have been heavily studied.[6] It is not clear that the reduction in infant mortality in the first half of the 20th century (which had a large effect on the rate of change in US life expectancy) or the stagnation of life expectancy in the 1960s, when the reckoning came for high rates of smoking in the 1940s and 1950s, offer us much guidance today.

A primary objective of health systems is to promote the health of the population. If this aim is to be achieved, we need to examine who is dying and of what. This will generally require studying individual death records. The work must shine light on the rise in premature deaths from drugs, alcohol, and suicide—three of the four causes that Woolf notes are causing midlife mortality to rise in the United States—as well as the decrease in progress against cardiovascular disease, which was the engine of US mortality decrease in the last third of the 20th century.[1,6]

We need to understand the mechanisms that lead to premature death. Some of this work has begun, with a focus on the role of education.[7–11] Case and Deaton highlighted growing educational gaps in mortality (all cause and by cause) for non-Hispanic Whites aged 45 to 54 years.[12] Our research since that time has focused on the clear difference in mortality outcomes throughout adulthood for Americans with and without a four-year college degree. Those with a four-year college degree saw all-cause mortality fall and adult life expectancy continue to increase before the COVID-19 pandemic, whereas those with less than a four-year college degree saw mortality increase and adult life expectancy fall for almost the entire decade before COVID-19.[13] Related work by Mackenbach et al. does not find any such pattern—of mortality moving in different directions by education—in any country in Western Europe but does document the same pattern in many countries in Eastern Europe following the collapse of the Soviet Union.[14] Comparisons of differences in the educational mortality gaps in the United States and Europe, and the causes behind them, may help us unearth underlying mechanisms.

Within education categories (four-year college degree vs no four-year college degree) racial divides in mortality between Black and White people narrowed by 70% between 1990 and 2018, whereas within race (Black, White) educational divides more than doubled for both racial groups.[14] Deaths of despair among non-Hispanic Black and Hispanic people began to rise after 2010. Like those for non-Hispanic White people, the increases are largely confined to those without a four-year college degree.

Additional research adds evidence of the importance of education in US mortality. Olfson et al., combining 3.4 million observations from the 2008 American Community Survey with the National Death Index from 2008 to 2015, found that the four-year college divide continues to predict death from drugs, alcohol, and suicide (analyzed separately or jointly) over this period, even with controls for race, sex, age, income, marital status, and labor market outcomes.[15] Rising deaths of despair among those without a four-year college degree suggest a growing mental health crisis for this group, and recent analyses find evidence of this. Blanchflower and Oswald, using data from the Behavioral Risk Factor Surveillance System, found that extreme distress (reporting that 30 of the last 30 days mental health was not good) doubled for adults without a four-year college degree in the period from 1993 to 2019.[16] The connection between extreme distress and addiction is argued by neurobiologists.[17]

Case and Deaton found that the US mortality gap between those with versus those without a four-year college degree has been rising for three decades for all-cause mortality and in each of 13 broad cause of death classifications.[18] This has occurred in causes of death that have been falling (cancer), rising (deaths of despair), or falling then rising (cardiovascular disease) and in causes of death in which initially those with a four-year college degree had higher mortality rates.

Such results do not make a lack of higher education causal in the higher mortality rates for those without a four-year college degree, but they do suggest that something related to education may hold a key to understanding what is ailing the United States. In midlife broadly defined (aged 25–64 years), those without a four-year college degree have seen labor force attachment and marriage rates fall precipitously. From Olfson et al. we have evidence that these are correlates of deaths of despair. Wage rates for men without a four-year college degree have been stagnant for 50 years and, again from Olfson et al., lower income is also a correlate of death from drugs, suicide, and alcohol. As noted by Link and Phelan, individual characteristics—like educational attainment—must be contextualized "by examining what put *people at risk of risks*."[19p80] Understanding the relationship in the United States between educational attainment and poor social and economic outcomes may greatly increase our ability to make sense of the mortality landscape that we face. AJPH

CORRESPONDENCE

Correspondence should be sent to Anne Case, 215 Robertson Hall, Princeton University, Princeton, NJ 08544 (e-mail: accase@princeton.edu). Reprints can be ordered at http://www.ajph.org by clicking the "Reprints" link.

PUBLICATION INFORMATION

Full Citation: Case A. Something related to education may hold the key to understanding what is ailing the United States. *Am J Public Health*. 2023;113(9):964–966.

Acceptance Date: June 25, 2023.

DOI: https://doi.org/10.2105/AJPH.2023.307375

ACKNOWLEDGMENTS

I gratefully acknowledge support from the National Institute of Aging through an award to the National Bureau of Economic Research (award R01AG062014).

I thank Angus Deaton for comments on an earlier draft.

CONFLICTS OF INTEREST

The author has no conflicts of interest to declare.

REFERENCES

1. Deaton A. *The Great Escape: Health, Wealth and the Origins of Inequality.* Princeton, NJ: Princeton University Press; 2013.
2. World Health Organization. Civil registration: why counting births and deaths is important. May 30, 2014. Available at: https://www.who.int/news-room/fact-sheets/detail/civil-registration-why-counting-births-and-deaths-is-important. Accessed June 30, 2023.
3. GBD 2016 Causes of Death Collaborators. Global, regional, and national age-sex specific mortality for 264 causes of death, 1980–2016: a systematic analysis for the Global Burden of Disease Study 2016. *Lancet.* 2017;390(10100):1151–1210. [Erratum in: *Lancet.* 2017;390(10106):e38]. https://doi.org/10.1016/S0140-6736(17)32152-9
4. Lopez AD, McLaughlin D, Richards N. Reducing ignorance about who dies of what: research and innovation to strengthen CRVS systems. *BMC Med.* 2020;18(1):1–6. https://doi.org/10.1186/s12916-020-01526-9
5. Coale AJ, Demeny P, Vaughan B. *Regional Model Life Tables and Stable Populations.* New York, NY: Academic Press; 1983.
6. Crimmins EM, Preston SH, Cohen B; Panel on Understanding Divergent Trends in Longevity in High-Income Countries, eds. *Explaining Divergent Levels of Longevity in High-Income Countries.* Washington, DC: National Academies Press; 2011.
7. Meara ER, Richards S, Cutler DM. The gap gets bigger: changes in mortality and life expectancy, by education, 1981–2000. *Health Aff (Millwood).* 2008;27(2):350–360. https://doi.org/10.1377/hlthaff.27.2.350
8. Olshansky SJ, Antonucci T, Berkman L, et al. Differences in life expectancy due to race and educational differences are widening and many may not catch up. *Health Aff (Millwood).* 2012;31(8):1803–1813. https://doi.org/10.1377/hlthaff.2011.0746
9. Geronimus AT, Bound J, Waidman TA, Rodriguez JM, Timpe B. Weathering, drugs, and whack-a-mole: fundamental and proximate causes of widening educational inequity in US life expectancy by sex and race, 1990–2015. *J Health Soc Behav.* 2019;60(2):222–239. https://doi.org/10.1177/0022146519849932
10. Sasson I, Hayward MD. Association between educational attainment and causes of death among White and Black US adults, 2010–2017. *JAMA.* 2019;322(8):756–763. https://doi.org/10.1001/jama.2019.11330
11. Case A, Deaton A. The great divide: education, despair, and death. *Annu Rev Econ.* 2022;14:1–21. https://doi.org/10.1146/annurev-economics-051520-015607
12. Case A, Deaton A. Rising morbidity and mortality in midlife among White non-Hispanic Americans in the 21st century. *Proc Natl Acad Sci U S A.* 2015;112(49):15078–15083. https://doi.org/10.1073/pnas.1518393112
13. Case A, Deaton A. Life expectancy in adulthood is falling for those without a BA degree, but as educational gaps have widened, racial gaps have narrowed. *Proc Natl Acad Sci U S A.* 2021;118(11):e2024777118. https://doi.org/10.1073/pnas.2024777118
14. Mackenbach JP, Valverde JR, Artnik B, et al. Trends in health inequalities in 27 European countries. *Proc Natl Acad Sci U S A.* 2018;115(25):6440–6445. https://doi.org/10.1073/pnas.1800028115
15. Olfson M, Cosgrove C, Altekruse SF, Wall MM, Blanco C. Deaths of despair: adults at high risk for death by suicide, poisoning, or chronic liver disease in the US. *Health Aff (Millwood).* 2021;40(3):505–512. https://doi.org/10.1377/hlthaff.2020.01573
16. Blanchflower DG, Oswald AJ. Trends in extreme distress in the United States, 1993–2019. *Am J Public Health.* 2020;110(10):1538–1544. https://doi.org/10.2105/AJPH.2020.305811
17. Koob GF, Powell P, White A. Addiction as a coping response: hyperkatifeia, deaths of despair, and COVID-19. *Am J Psychiatry.* 2020;177(11):1031–1037. https://doi.org/10.1176/appi.ajp.2020.20091375
18. Case A, Deaton A. *Accounting for the Widening Mortality Gap Between Adult Americans With and Without a BA.* Cambridge, MA: National Bureau of Economic Research; 2023. NBER working paper no. 31236.
19. Link BG, Phelan J. Social conditions as fundamental causes of disease. *J Health Soc Behav.* 1995;(spec no):80–94.

The Gap Between US and Best Practice Life Expectancy Is Increasing

José Manuel Aburto, PhD, and Serena Vigezzi, MSc

ABOUT THE AUTHORS

José Manuel Aburto is with the Department of Population Health, London School of Hygiene and Tropical Medicine, London, UK, and the Leverhulme Centre for Demographic Science, University of Oxford, Oxford, UK. Both authors are with the Interdisciplinary Centre on Population Dynamics, University of Southern Denmark, Odense.

See also US Life Expectancy, pp. 952–980.

Period life expectancy at birth is widely used as an indicator of population health. It summarizes the mortality profile as the average number of years a synthetic cohort of newborns is expected to live if they experience the death rates observed in a given year throughout their lives.[1] It is not a forecast nor a projection of any real individual's lifespan, although its name may suggest otherwise. Nevertheless, life expectancy allows reliable comparisons over time and between populations, as it is not affected by population size and age structure. Using demographic methods, it is also possible to disentangle which ages or causes of death account for changes over time in life expectancy.

Life expectancy in the United States increased in the second half of the 20th century (from 68.1 years in 1950 to 76.8 years in 2000) but remained below the levels of other high-income countries. In the decade preceding the COVID-19 pandemic, it stagnated and even decreased.[1] Several health-related factors explain the underperformance of US life expectancy and the widening gap with other high-income countries. These include a higher rate of smoking-related mortality,[2] a high prevalence of obesity,[3] a lack of improvements in mortality from cardiovascular diseases,[4] and the unprecedented increase in deaths from suicide and drug and alcohol use.[5] The US disadvantage in health and mortality was further aggravated during the COVID-19 pandemic. In 2020, the United States suffered the largest loss in life expectancy among high-income countries (2.2 years),[1] with sizable ethnic/racial and geographic differences in these losses.[6,7] In 2021, the detrimental consequences of the pandemic continued. Although most Western European countries experienced improvements in mortality in 2021 compared to 2020, in the United States, life expectancy decreased by a further seven months.[8]

In this issue of *AJPH*, Woolf (p. 970) provides another perspective for analyzing life expectancy trends in the United States as a whole and its states individually. He compares observed values since the 1930s to the best practice life expectancy, defined as the highest life expectancy observed among countries worldwide in a given year. This indicator steadily increased by three months per year from 1840 to 2000.[9] By contrast to the best practice trend, Woolf shows that the rate of life expectancy increase in the United States has varied substantially since 1950. Periods of more rapid increase in the early 1950s and the late 1970s were followed by sharp slowdowns, stagnation since 2010, and decrease during the COVID-19 pandemic. During this period, the gap between US and best practice life expectancy increased from 3.5 years in 1950 to 6.1 years in 2019 and 8.3 in 2021. Compared with other countries with more than half a million inhabitants, US life expectancy lost ground by falling from being the 12th highest in 1950 to the 40th in 2019. The United States underperformed not only compared with other wealthy countries, as has been widely reported, but also compared with 20 middle-income countries, especially since the mid-1970s. A salient point of Woolf's study is the analysis of life expectancy by US state, which shows large variation in life expectancy levels and trends. The slowest increases in life expectancy happened in South Central states and the Midwest, which together account for more than half of US states that suffered decreases in life expectancy in the decade before the pandemic.

Comparisons with best practice life expectancy can be informative for quantifying potential gains in life expectancy and can offer a realistic benchmark in mortality forecasting. There are, however, some limitations to this approach. Best practice life expectancy is a composite indicator, in that the best practice country can differ from year to year, creating an ever-changing reference. For example, Norway and Japan held the best practice life expectancy in 1977 and 1978, respectively. These countries have their own, distinctive epidemiological profile, which raises

AJPH September 2023, Vol 113, No. 9

questions of comparability with the United States but also between countries that hold the best practice life expectancy in different years. Whether the United States could reach best practice life expectancy might depend on factors that may be impossible or undesirable to change, such as environmental conditions or cultural aspects.

Even though the referenced data sets are stratified by age and sex, these two fundamental demographic dimensions were not considered in Woolf's analysis. Investigating the extent to which different ages can account for the US disadvantage in life expectancy or whether this gap is larger for females than males is essential to understand from a public health perspective to assess whether everyone benefits equally from mortality improvements. The rapid decrease of infectious diseases in the early 20th century benefited young females more than males,[10] and in general females live longer than males because of social risk factors (e.g., violent behavior), biological traits, and genetic differences, among other reasons.

Using standard decomposition analysis applied to the Human Mortality Database, it is easy to show that ages that explain the gap between US and best practice life expectancy have changed over time and are different between sexes (Figure 1). Up to the late 1970s, the gap between US and best practice life expectancy was mainly driven by mortality disadvantage for those younger than 50 years, with infant mortality contributing substantially (around a third for females). From the 1990s, contributions from those older than 50 years dominated, whereas age groups between 20 and 60 years contributed approximately 50% to the gap with best practice life expectancy in 2015 and 2020.

Beyond age, sex, and geographical differences, salient features of the historic US disadvantage are the stark and persistent social inequalities that pattern it. Most racial/ethnic minorities experience higher death rates than non-Hispanic White people throughout their lives.[6] Although this disadvantage decreased during most of the 20th and the beginning of the 21st century, it has remained large, even surpassing the impact of COVID-19 on non-Hispanic White people's life expectancy.[1] This heterogeneity stems in part from a different distribution of causes of death. In the 2010s, non-Hispanic White people were more severely affected by the increase in suicides and accidental poisonings. However, Black people,

AJPH September 2023, Vol 113, No. 9

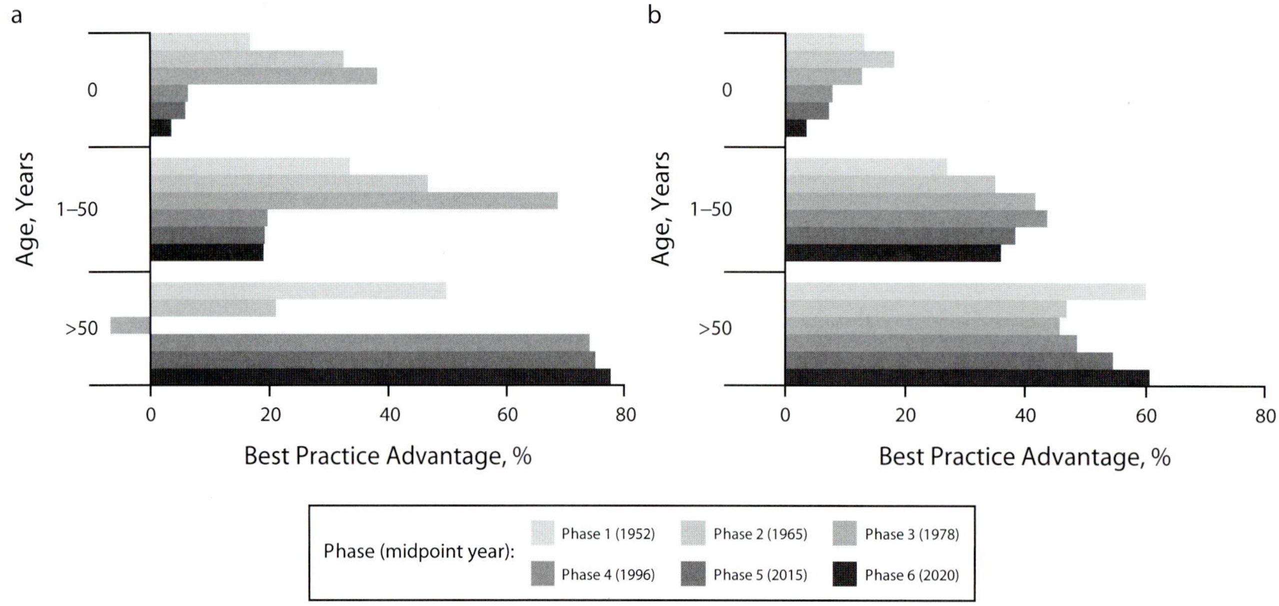

FIGURE 1— Decomposition Into 3 Age Groups of the Life Expectancy Gap Between the United States and the Best Practice Country at the Midpoint Year of Every Phase Identified by Woolf, by (a) Females and (b) Males: 1952, 1965, 1978, 1996, 2015, and 2020

Note. Positive values indicate that the mortality difference in that age group advantaged the best practice country, and negative values indicate age groups for which the United States had lower mortality rates than the best practice country.
Source. See Woolf, in this issue of *AJPH*, p. 970.

especially men, were much more affected by homicides and have historically had higher rates of cardiovascular mortality, whereas Hispanic people have had high alcohol-related mortality.[11] In 2020, higher mortality from COVID-19 aggravated the Black disadvantage and reduced the mortality advantage that Hispanic people had so far maintained, overall improving non-Hispanic White people's relative position.[6] Similarly, some of the least educated groups experienced stagnation and even a decrease in life expectancy as early as the 1990s, whereas the most educated populations kept improving.[12]

Woolf's work confirms the wide-ranging disadvantage of the United States with respect to other countries. Future work should continue to examine the impact of existing, and potentially growing, social inequalities as well as the long-term consequences of the social and economic disruptions brought about by the pandemic on population health to ultimately inform public health policy. AJPH

CORRESPONDENCE

Correspondence should be sent to José Manuel Aburto, Keppel St, London WC1E 7HT, UK (e-mail: jose.aburto@lshtm.ac.uk). Reprints can be ordered at http://www.ajph.org by clicking the "Reprints" link.

PUBLICATION INFORMATION

Full Citation: Aburto JM, Vigezzi S. The gap between US and best practice life expectancy is increasing. *Am J Public Health*. 2023;113(9): 967–969.

Acceptance Date: April 18, 2023.

DOI: https://doi.org/10.2105/AJPH.2023.307332

CONTRIBUTORS

The authors contributed equally to this editorial.

ACKNOWLEDGMENTS

J. M. Aburto was supported by the European Union Horizon 2020 research and innovation programme (Marie Sklodowska-Curie grant 896821) and the ROCKWOOL Foundation (Excess Deaths grant).

The authors thank Ridhi Kashyap for comments and suggestions on this editorial.

CONFLICTS OF INTEREST

The authors have no conflicts of interest to declare.

REFERENCES

1. Schöley J, Aburto JM, Kashnitsky I, et al. Life expectancy changes since COVID-19. *Nat Hum Behav.* 2022;6(12):1649–1659. https://doi.org/10.1038/s41562-022-01450-3
2. Glei DA, Lee C, Weinstein M. Socioeconomic disparities in U.S. mortality: the role of smoking and alcohol/drug abuse. *SSM Popul Health.* 2020;12:100699. https://doi.org/10.1016/j.ssmph.2020.100699
3. Preston SH, Stokes A. Contribution of obesity to international differences in life expectancy. *Am J Public Health.* 2011;101(11):2137–2143. https://doi.org/10.2105/AJPH.2011.300219
4. Mehta NK, Abrams LR, Myrskylä M. US life expectancy stalls due to cardiovascular disease, not drug deaths. *Proc Natl Acad Sci U S A.* 2020;117(13):6998–7000. https://doi.org/10.1073/pnas.1920391117
5. Tilstra AM, Simon DH, Masters RK. Trends in "deaths of despair" among working-aged White and Black Americans, 1990–2017. *Am J Epidemiol.* 2021;190(9):1751–1759. https://doi.org/10.1093/aje/kwab088
6. Aburto JM, Tilstra AM, Floridi G, Dowd JB. Significant impacts of the COVID-19 pandemic on race/ethnic differences in US mortality. *Proc Natl Acad Sci U S A.* 2022;119(35):e2205813119. https://doi.org/10.1073/pnas.2205813119
7. Stokes AC, Lundberg DJ, Elo IT, Hempstead K, Bor J, Preston SH. COVID-19 and excess mortality in the United States: a county-level analysis. *PLoS Med.* 2021;18(5):e1003571. https://doi.org/10.1371/journal.pmed.1003571
8. Andrasfay T, Goldman N. Reductions in US life expectancy during the COVID-19 pandemic by race and ethnicity: is 2021 a repetition of 2020? *medRxiv* [Preprint July 19, 2022; Update in *PLoS One*. 2022;17(8):e0272973]. https://doi.org/10.1101/2021.10.17.21265117
9. Oeppen J, Vaupel JW. Demography. Broken limits to life expectancy. *Science.* 2002;296(5570):1029–1031. https://doi.org/10.1126/science.1069675
10. Goldin C, Lleras-Muney A. XX > XY?: the changing female advantage in life expectancy. *J Health Econ.* 2019;67:102224. https://doi.org/10.1016/j.jhealeco.2019.102224
11. Harper S, Riddell CA, King NB. Declining life expectancy in the United States: missing the trees for the forest. *Annu Rev Public Health.* 2021;42:381–403. https://doi.org/10.1146/annurev-publhealth-082619-104231
12. Sasson I. Trends in life expectancy and lifespan variation by educational attainment: United States, 1990–2010. *Demography.* 2016;53(2):269–293. https://doi.org/10.1007/s13524-015-0453-7

Falling Behind: The Growing Gap in Life Expectancy Between the United States and Other Countries, 1933–2021

Steven H. Woolf, MD, MPH

See also US Life Expectancy, pp. 952–980.

Objectives. To document the evolution of the US life expectancy disadvantage and regional variation across the US states.

Methods. I obtained life expectancy estimates in 2022 from the United Nations, the Human Mortality Database, and the US Mortality Database, and calculated changes in growth rates, US global position (rank), and state-level trends.

Results. Increases in US life expectancy slowed from 1950 to 1954 (0.21 years/annum) and 1955 to 1973 (0.10 years/annum), accelerated from 1974 to 1982 (0.34 years/annum), and progressively deteriorated from 1983 to 2009 (0.15 years/annum), 2010 to 2019 (0.06 years/annum), and 2020 to 2021 (–0.97 years/annum). Other countries experienced faster growth in each phase except 1974 to 1982. During 1933 to 2021, 56 countries on 6 continents surpassed US life expectancy. Growth in US life expectancy was slowest in Midwest and South Central states.

Conclusions. The US life expectancy disadvantage began in the 1950s and has steadily worsened over the past 4 decades. Dozens of globally diverse countries have outperformed the United States. Causal factors appear to have been concentrated in the Midwest and South.

Public Health Implications. Policies that differentiate the United States from other countries and circumstances associated with the Midwest and South may have contributed. (*Am J Public Health*. 2023;113(9):970–980. https://doi.org/10.2105/AJPH.2023.307310)

AJPH September 2023, Vol 113, No. 9

The United States suffers from a health disadvantage: the US population experiences poorer health than populations in other countries, and the disadvantage has grown over time.[1] One component of this phenomenon is the US life expectancy disadvantage: survival in the developed world has increased over the past century, but growth in US life expectancy has not kept pace with that of other industrialized countries. The gap with other countries widened dramatically after 2010, when life expectancy plateaued in the United States but continued increasing elsewhere.[2]

A recent demonstration of the US health disadvantage occurred during the COVID-19 pandemic, when the United States experienced more COVID-19 deaths than any other country and among the highest per capita death rates.[3] US life expectancy decreased by 2.1 years between 2019 and 2021, the largest decrease in a century.[2–4] Other high-income countries experienced smaller decreases in life expectancy during the pandemic, widening the gap to historic levels.[2]

The US life expectancy disadvantage began decades ago but exactly when remains unclear. Studies typically date the onset to the 1980s or 1990s, raising intriguing research questions about events in history that might explain this timing. Researchers usually measure the US life expectancy gap in reference to "peer countries," typically selecting high-income—and largely Western European or Anglo-Saxon—countries as the comparison group.[1,5–8] The implicit assumption is that less affluent or developing countries are unlikely to outperform the United States and cannot serve as a benchmark for documenting a US disadvantage. The validity of either assumption—that only high-income countries surpassed the United States and that the phenomenon began in the 1980s to 1990s—is unclear.

Clarifying the timing and geographic scale of the US life expectancy disadvantage is important groundwork for investigating potential causes. For example, knowing the years when changes occurred in the slope—the rate of change in US life expectancy—is a prerequisite for future studies of period and cohort effects. Comparing this "growth rate" with the slope in comparison countries would clarify when and how the US trajectory diverged. Furthermore, examining how life expectancy trends varied across the country can identify states where adverse life expectancy trends were geographically concentrated.

Several databases could help answer these questions but have not been examined with these aims. For example, the Population Division of the UN Department of Economic and Social Affairs has estimated life expectancy for 237 countries (and other geographic areas) for 1950 to 2021.[9] The Human Mortality Database—maintained by the University of California, Berkeley, the Max Planck Institute for Demographic Research in Germany, and the French Institute for Demographic Studies—provides life expectancy estimates for more than 40 countries, including 22 populous countries with data from before 1950.[10] Finally, the University of California, Berkeley maintains the US Mortality Database, which provides life tables for 1959 to 2020 for the 50 US states, the District of Columbia, and US Census Bureau regions.[11]

In this study, I merged data from these 3 sources to document the history and geographic progression of the US life expectancy disadvantage over 8 decades, analyzing a longer period than most studies have considered and widening the scope beyond high-income countries. The study addressed 4 research questions (see subquestions in Table A, available as a supplement to the online version of this article at http://www.ajph.org):

1. Over the observation period, how many countries achieved higher life expectancy than the United States, when, and for how long?
2. How did the position (rank) of the United States relative to other countries change over time?
3. How did the slope (rate of increase in life expectancy) vary in the United States, and when did it diverge from the average slope in other countries?
4. How did life expectancy in the 50 states compare with other countries, and which states made the greatest contributions to adverse US life expectancy trends?

METHODS

I focused the analysis on countries that "surpassed" the United States (achieved higher life expectancy) in at least 1 year of the observation period. Because life expectancy estimates can be unstable for small populations, I examined data only for "populous" countries, defined here as those with populations greater than 500 000 (based on UN data[9]).

Data Sources

I obtained life expectancy estimates for the period before 1950 from the Human Mortality Database. That database provides pre-1950 life expectancy estimates for the United States, beginning in 1933; beginning earlier in 18 other countries, including Sweden (1751–), France (1816–), Denmark (1835–), Iceland (1838–), Belgium (1841–), Norway (1846–), the Netherlands (1850–), Scotland (1855–), Italy (1872–), Switzerland (1876–), Finland (1878–), Spain (1908–), Australia (1921–), Canada (1921–), the United Kingdom (1922–), and Northern Ireland (1922–); and beginning later in 4 countries: Portugal (1940–), Bulgaria (1947–), Japan (1947–), and New Zealand (1948–).

I extracted life expectancy estimates for the United States and 236 other countries for the period of 1950 to 2021 from the July 2022 UN Population Division data release.[9] The UN derived these estimates from official life tables, registered deaths, and modeling methods described elsewhere.[12,13] The UN reported life expectancy estimates for countries and areas as defined in the statistical codes of the UN Secretariat,[14] which included territories (e.g., Puerto Rico) and some areas that are not universally recognized as countries (e.g., Taiwan, Hong Kong, Macao). The UN provided estimates for countries under their current names (e.g., Czechia, Slovenia) and for previous years when those areas were circumscribed in other countries (e.g., Czechoslovakia, Yugoslavia). They combined preunification (pre-1990) data for East and West Germany. I used World Bank sources to classify the income status of countries and to designate "centrally planned," or Communist, economies.[15,16]

I obtained life expectancy estimates for US states for 1959 to 2019 from the US Mortality Database.[11]

Data Analysis

I grouped countries by continent[17] and US states by US Census Bureau regions (n = 4) and divisions (n = 9).[18] I determined the period of "dominance" (the calendar years when a country's life expectancy exceeded US life expectancy), total years of dominance during 1950 to 2021, and the country's income status at the time of dominance.

For each year, I examined the gap between US life expectancy and that of the populous country with the highest life expectancy (Norway in 1950–1962 and 1976–1977, Sweden in 1963 and 1965–1975, the Netherlands in 1964, Japan in 1978–2007, Macao in 2008–2010, and Hong Kong in 2011–2021). For the period 1959 to 2019, I compared estimates of life expectancy by state from the US Mortality Database and by country from UN data to determine where states would rank if they were countries (excluding the United States and other states when determining rankings). For context, I identified 4 "adjacent" populous countries with the most comparable life expectancy: 2 higher and 2 lower. I included countries that never surpassed the United States only for this contextual analysis.

To examine temporal trends in the United States and other populous countries, I calculated year-over-year absolute changes in life expectancy and mean year-over-year changes for the entire 70-year period (1950–2021), for each decade, and for 6 periods (phases) with distinctly different growth rates in US life expectancy. For all 4 measures (yearly changes and mean changes for 1950–2021 and each decade and phase), I also calculated the median value for mean changes in life expectancy among populous countries. In calculations of slopes and rankings, I excluded values for countries with populations below 500 000 during the years of analysis. Because estimates from the UN and US Mortality Database began with 1950 and 1959, respectively, measures of annual increases began with 1951 and 1960.

RESULTS

Growth in US life expectancy during 1950 to 2021 (Figure 1a) occurred in 6 phases with distinctly different slopes (growth rates): phase 1 (1950–1954), a period of brisk growth (0.21 years/annum); phase 2 (1955–1973), when growth slowed by half (0.10 years/annum); phase 3 (1974–1982), when the growth rate rebounded (0.34 years/annum); phase 4 (1983–2009), when growth slowed by half (0.15 years/annum) and remained slow for more than 2 decades; phase 5 (2010–2019), when life expectancy plateaued (0.06 years/annum); and phase 6 (2020–2021), when life expectancy decreased sharply (–0.97 years/annum) during the COVID-19 pandemic.

Life Expectancy

In 1933 (when US estimates first appear in the Human Mortality Database), US life expectancy ranked 8th highest among 16 populous countries, behind the Netherlands, Norway, Australia, Sweden, Denmark, Switzerland, and Canada. These countries, along with the United Kingdom, generally maintained higher life expectancy than the United States from the 1930s through World War II and the late 1940s.

In 1950, US life expectancy ranked 12th highest among populous countries in the UN database, and the gap with the top performer was 3.5 years (Figure 1b). When the US growth rate slowed in phase 2 (1955–1973), 19 countries surpassed the United States. By 1968, the US rank had fallen to 29th. The United States rebounded temporarily in the 1970s, recovering much of these losses; in 1976, US life expectancy ranked 13th among populous countries. However, the United States began losing ground to other countries in the early 1980s; between 1983 and 2009, US ranking among populous countries fell from 15th to 32nd, and the life expectancy gap with the top performer rose from 2.6 years to 4.7 years (Table B, available as a supplement to the online version of this article at http://www.ajph.org). During 2010 to 2019, when US life expectancy plateaued, 7 more populous countries surpassed the United States.

By 2019, the eve of the COVID-19 pandemic, US life expectancy ranked 40th among populous countries—lower than in Albania and Lebanon—and the life expectancy gap with the top performer was 6.1 years. Large decreases in US life expectancy during the pandemic enabled 6 more populous countries to surpass the United States. In 2020, US life expectancy ranked 46th among populous countries, and the gap reached 7.8 years.

Life Expectancy Growth Rates

US ranking decreased because other populous countries averaged larger annual increases in life expectancy in 49 of the 70 years studied. As detailed elsewhere (Table C, available as a supplement to the online version of this article at http://www.ajph.org), the mean US growth rate was lower than median growth in other populous countries when analyzed on multiple measures: for the entire 7-decade period (1951–2021), in each individual decade but the 1970s, and in each phase except phase 3 (1974–1982). The US growth rate was outperformed by 48 populous countries during phase 4 (1983–2009) and by all populous countries but Cuba (n = 56) during phase 5 (2010–2019). Although growth slowed across many countries during phase 5,

AJPH September 2023, Vol 113, No. 9

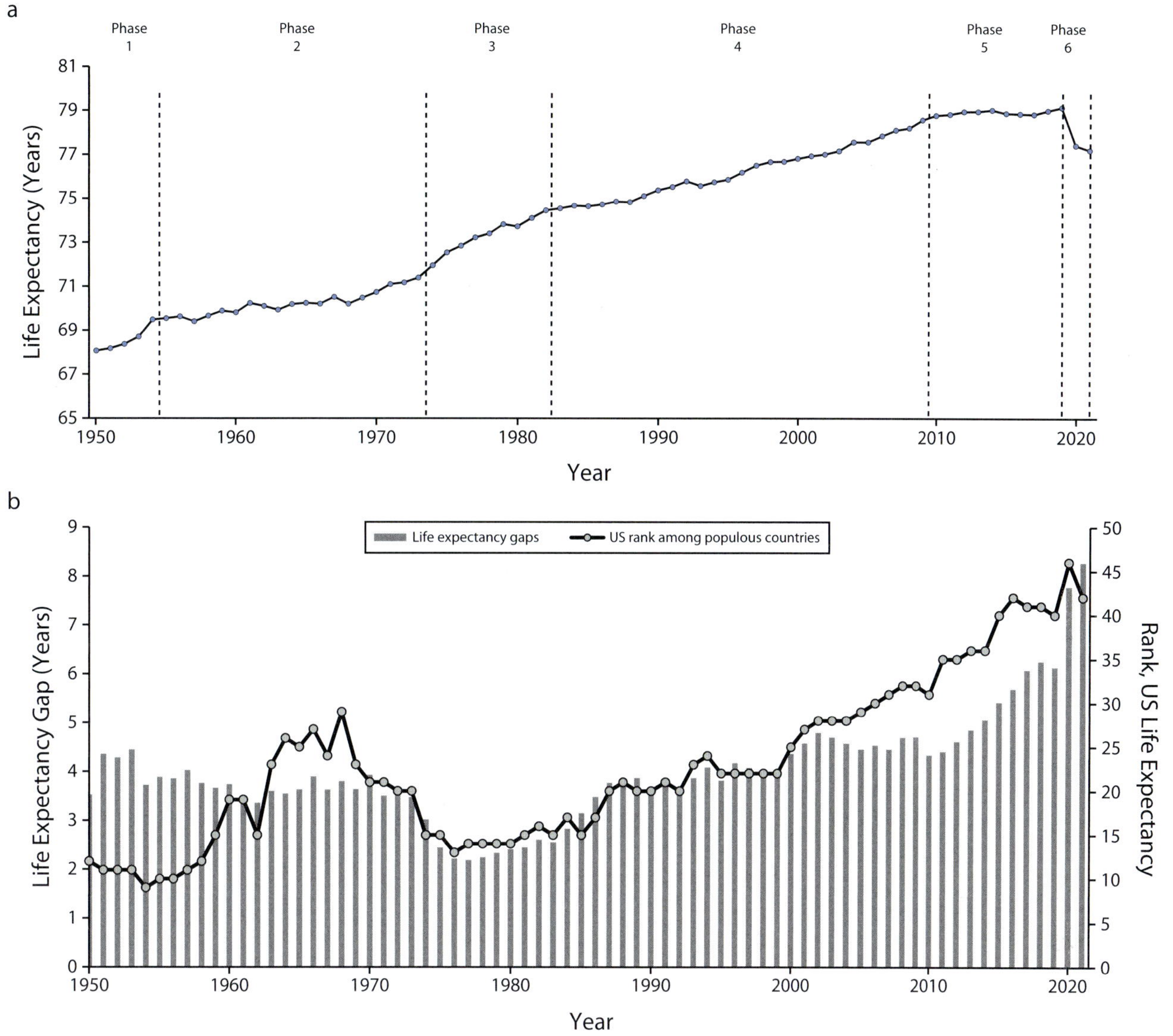

FIGURE 1— Change Over Time in (a) US Life Expectancy and (b) US Life Expectancy Gap and Rank Relative to Populous Countries (Population > 500 000): 1950–2021

Note. Phase 1 = 1950–1954; phase 2 = 1955–1973; phase 3 = 1974–1982; phase 4 = 1983–2009; phase 5 = 2010–2019; phase 6 = 2020–2021. Bars plot the difference in life expectancy between the United States and the populous country (population > 500 000) with the highest life expectancy in the given year. The country with the highest life expectancy was Norway in 1950–1962 and 1976–1977, Sweden in 1963 and 1965–1975, the Netherlands in 1964, Japan in 1978–2007, Macao in 2008–2010, and Hong Kong in 2011–2021. The line graph plots US rank relative to other populous countries, with higher rank denoting lower US life expectancy.
Source. Author's calculations based on UN data.[9]

the median pace in populous countries (0.18 years/annum) was still triple that of the United States (0.06 years/annum), and other countries experienced smaller losses in life expectancy during phase 6 (COVID-19 pandemic).

Between 1933 and 2021, 56 populous countries on multiple continents achieved higher life expectancy than the United States (Figure 2; Figure A and Table D, available as a supplement to the online version of this article at http://www.ajph.org). Before 1950, most populous countries that outperformed the United States were in Northern and Western Europe, with a few exceptions (Australia, Canada, Israel, Latvia, New Zealand). However, in the 1950s and 1960s, Southern European (e.g., Greece, Italy, Spain) and additional Western European countries (e.g., Austria, France, Belgium, Germany, Ireland) surpassed the United States, as did several Eastern

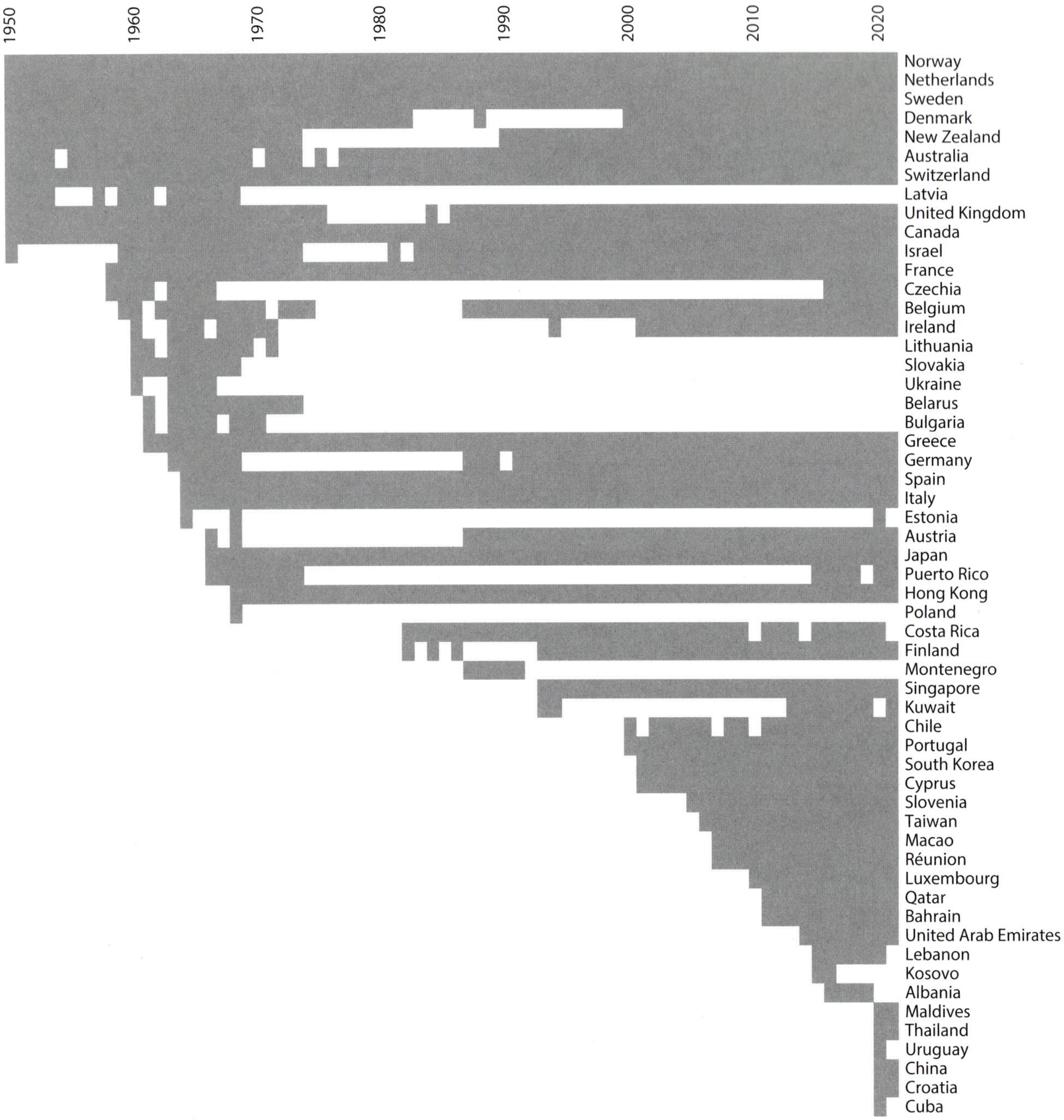

FIGURE 2— Populous Countries That Achieved Higher Life Expectancy Than the United States and Calendar Years of Dominance: 1950–2021

Note. Shaded bars depict the calendar years during which populous countries (populations > 500 000) experienced higher life expectancy than the United States; interruptions in bars reflect periods when the United States recovered its advantage (experienced higher life expectancy). A more detailed version of this figure (Figure A, available as a supplement to the online version of this article at http://www.ajph.org) includes each country's ranking, by year, among populous countries, showing how the relative position of countries surpassing the United States progressed over time.
Source. Author's calculations based on UN data.[9]

Bloc countries (e.g., Belarus, Bulgaria, Czechoslovakia, Lithuania, Ukraine). Asian countries also surpassed the United States, beginning with Japan and Hong Kong in the 1960s and followed by other East Asian countries in the 1990s and beyond. The United States was also surpassed by several Eastern European countries after 2000 and by Middle Eastern states, beginning with Kuwait in the 1990s and followed by Bahrain, Qatar, United Arab

AJPH September 2023, Vol 113, No. 9

Emirates, and Lebanon after 2010. US life expectancy was surpassed by 11 middle-income and 9 Communist countries. Seventeen countries outperformed the United States for more than 50 years.

State Contribution to US Changes

In 1959, when US Mortality Database estimates begin, Kansas and South Carolina had the nation's highest and lowest life expectancy, respectively. Were these states countries, they would have ranked 5th and 34th among the world's populous countries. Populous countries closest in life expectancy ("adjacent" countries) to Kansas were the Netherlands and Denmark (next highest life expectancy) and Switzerland and the United Kingdom (next lowest), whereas countries adjacent to South Carolina were Hungary and Bulgaria (higher) and Poland and Hong Kong (lower). Over the ensuing 60 years, US states experienced a diminished global position and greater divergence in life expectancy. By 2019, the state with the highest life expectancy, Hawaii, ranked 22nd—adjacent to Austria and Finland (higher) and the United Kingdom and Portugal (lower)—whereas the state with the lowest life expectancy, Mississippi, ranked 79th, adjacent to Mauritius and Bulgaria (higher) and Ukraine and Morocco (lower).

Increases in life expectancy between 1959 and 2019 differed across the 50 states (Table 1; Table E, available as a supplement to the online version of this article at http://www.ajph.org). Growth rates were generally highest in the Northeast (US Census divisions 1–2) and West (divisions 8–9) and lowest in South Central states (US Census divisions 6–7) and the Midwest (divisions 3–4), especially during phases 4 and 5 (Figure 3). In phases 3 to 5, strong growth occurred in the Atlantic coastal states of division 5 (from Delaware to Florida), but growth rates were low in West Virginia, that division's 1 inland state. The Midwest experienced the lowest growth rates in phases 2 and 4 and accounted for more than half of the 17 states that experienced negative growth (i.e., decreases) in phase 5 (Table 1). All 50 states contributed to the national decline in phases 4 and 5: no state—even states with the highest growth rates—outperformed the US growth rate of the previous phase. Nor did any state match the median growth of populous countries in phases 2, 4, and 5 (except Hawaii and Nevada in phase 2). Patterns reversed during the US rebound in phase 3, when all states but Oklahoma outpaced median growth in populous countries.

DISCUSSION

Studies of the US health disadvantage typically make comparisons with 15 to 30 high-income countries, consisting mostly of British Commonwealth (e.g., United Kingdom, Australia, Canada) and Western European "peer countries."[1,2,5–8] I found that the 56 countries that outperformed the United States spanned the globe, from East Asia to Central and South America, Eastern Europe, and the Middle East. Moreover, 20 were middle-income or Communist countries when they surpassed the United States. Some developing countries experienced spectacular increases in life expectancy and now rank among the healthiest in the world. For example, in 1959, Hong Kong had lower life expectancy than South Carolina but by 2011 had the world's highest life expectancy.

A 2013 National Research Council report explored 5 domains that might explain the US health disadvantage—health systems, individual behaviors, socioeconomic factors, the environment, and policies and social values—and with each domain found distinctive US characteristics that might contribute to poorer health.[1] Potential contributors included not only downstream, proximal factors such as obesity, substance abuse, and deficiencies in the US health care system but also upstream, macrostructural factors such as US policies. For example, countries with better health outcomes typically offer more generous social welfare and income support programs and enforce stronger regulations to protect public health and safety.[19,20]

Explanations for the US life expectancy disadvantage must account for its timing—when in US history it began and why growth rates changed over particular years. Previous studies dated the onset to the 1980s or 1990s, prompting speculation about the roles of the obesity epidemic, Reagan era policies, and the opioid crisis that followed the 1996 licensing of OxyContin.[7] However, I found that growth in US life expectancy began slowing as early as phase 2 (1955–1973), allowing 3 countries in the late 1950s and 16 countries in the 1960s to surpass the United States. The rebound in phase 3 (1974–1982) temporarily halted further losses, but the slowing that followed in phase 4 (1983–2009) allowed the United States to be surpassed by 3 countries in the 1980s, 2 countries in the 1990s, and 8 countries in the 2000s.

Understanding the complex reasons for these changes in slope will require further research. Some explanations[6,7,21,22] have emerged for phase 5 (2010–2019), the decade in which US life expectancy plateaued, allowing 7 more countries to surpass the United States. A 2021 report by the National Academies of Science,

TABLE 1— Yearly Change in Life Expectancy in US States, United States (Total), and Populous Countries: 1960–2019 and Phases 2–5

Location	Increases in Life Expectancy (Years/Annum), by Period				
	1960–2019	Phase 2 (1960–1973)	Phase 3 (1974–1982)	Phase 4 (1983–2009)	Phase 5 (2010–2019)
Populous countries[a] (median)	0.21	0.20	0.24	0.23	0.18
United States[b] (mean)	0.15	0.11	0.34	0.15	0.06
Region 1: Northeast					
Division 1: New England					
Connecticut	0.16	0.15	0.26	0.18	0.03
Massachusetts	0.17	0.12	0.34	0.17	0.06
Maine	0.15	0.15	0.38	0.14	−0.05
New Hampshire	0.16	0.13	0.36	0.17	−0.04
Rhode Island	0.16	0.14	0.35	0.15	0.03
Vermont	0.16	0.13	0.33	0.19	−0.02
Division 2: Mid-Atlantic					
New Jersey	0.18	0.13	0.29	0.20	0.06
New York	0.19	0.14	0.29	0.22	0.13
Pennsylvania	0.15	0.12	0.35	0.15	0.04
Region 2: Midwest					
Division 3: East North Central					
Illinois	0.16	0.08	0.37	0.17	0.08
Indiana	0.11	0.06	0.36	0.11	−0.02
Michigan	0.14	0.06	0.33	0.15	0.02
Ohio	0.12	0.08	0.33	0.12	−0.04
Wisconsin	0.14	0.14	0.31	0.14	−0.04
Division 4: West North Central					
Iowa	0.12	0.10	0.34	0.12	−0.03
Kansas	0.11	0.08	0.30	0.10	−0.01
Minnesota	0.15	0.14	0.34	0.15	−0.002
Missouri	0.11	0.06	0.35	0.11	0.00
Nebraska	0.13	0.11	0.29	0.13	−0.01
North Dakota	0.13	0.11	0.38	0.10	−0.01
South Dakota	0.13	0.14	0.29	0.14	−0.05
Region 3: South					
Division 5: South Atlantic					
Delaware	0.15	0.10	0.29	0.17	0.04
Florida	0.16	0.07	0.39	0.15	0.11
Georgia	0.17	0.08	0.44	0.15	0.08
Maryland	0.17	0.06	0.35	0.11	0.00
North Carolina	0.16	0.08	0.45	0.14	0.05
South Carolina	0.18	0.13	0.51	0.15	0.04
Virginia	0.18	0.14	0.39	0.17	0.08
West Virginia	0.09	0.06	0.36	0.07	−0.03
Division 6: East South Central					
Alabama	0.12	0.10	0.41	0.07	0.03
Kentucky	0.10	0.05	0.34	0.08	−0.003

Continued

TABLE 1— Continued

	Increases in Life Expectancy (Years/Annum), by Period				
Location	1960–2019	Phase 2 (1960–1973)	Phase 3 (1974–1982)	Phase 4 (1983–2009)	Phase 5 (2010–2019)
Mississippi	0.11	0.09	0.40	0.08	−0.02
Tennessee	0.11	0.07	0.38	0.08	−0.02
Division 7: West South Central					
Arkansas	0.10	0.05	0.35	0.06	0.04
Louisiana	0.13	0.08	0.34	0.12	0.07
Oklahoma	0.08	0.06	0.20	0.07	0.05
Texas	0.14	0.05	0.34	0.15	0.09
Region 4: West					
Division 8: Mountain					
Arizona	0.17	0.18	0.36	0.14	0.07
Colorado	0.16	0.13	0.35	0.14	0.07
Idaho	0.14	0.12	0.33	0.14	0.03
Montana	0.16	0.14	0.39	0.13	0.05
Nevada	0.18	0.20	0.29	0.16	0.09
New Mexico	0.13	0.09	0.43	0.12	−0.05
Utah	0.14	0.12	0.31	0.14	0.01
Wyoming	0.14	0.08	0.40	0.12	0.04
Division 9: Pacific					
Alaska	0.16	0.12	0.35	0.16	0.07
California	0.17	0.10	0.28	0.19	0.12
Hawaii	0.17	0.25	0.30	0.11	0.11
Oregon	0.15	0.14	0.35	0.13	0.06
Washington	0.16	0.13	0.36	0.14	0.07

Source. Author's calculations based on US Mortality Database[11] and UN[9] data. The table omits data on changes in life expectancy during phase 1 and early phase 2 (1955–1958), for which state-level life expectancy estimates were unavailable in the US Mortality Database.

[a]Populations of > 500 000. Values for 10 countries were included only for years in which their populations exceeded 500 000; these included Bahrain (1990–), Cyprus (1953–), Macao (2007–), Kuwait (1966–), Luxembourg (2010–), Maldives (2020–), Montenegro (1965–), Qatar (1995–), Réunion (1974–), and United Arab Emirates (1975–).
[b]State means are presented by US Census Bureau regions and divisions.[18]

Engineering, and Medicine attributed the stagnation in US life expectancy to an increase in mortality rates in midlife (25–64 years). This increase, which no other country experienced, was caused primarily by US deaths from drug overdoses, alcohol-related causes, suicides, and cardiometabolic diseases.[7]

By 2019, the eve of the COVID-19 pandemic, 39 populous countries had higher life expectancy than did the United States. The gap with Hong Kong, which had the world's highest life expectancy, was 6.1 years. Life expectancy in some US states was lower than in developing countries. In 2019, life expectancy in West Virginia and Mississippi was lower than in the State of Palestine. The large decrease in US life expectancy that occurred during the COVID-19 pandemic—larger than in all countries but Bulgaria and Slovakia[23]—enabled 6 more countries to surpass the United States. By 2021, the gap with Hong Kong had reached 8.3 years.

Limitations

Limitations of this study include the reliance on life expectancy estimates from the UN Population Division and US Mortality Database, which, although validated,[12,24] are subject to errors that could potentially skew rankings and year-over-year changes. The inclusion of territories and countries with contested legal status could also affect rankings. The method used to define phases 1 to 5 may be less precise than determining

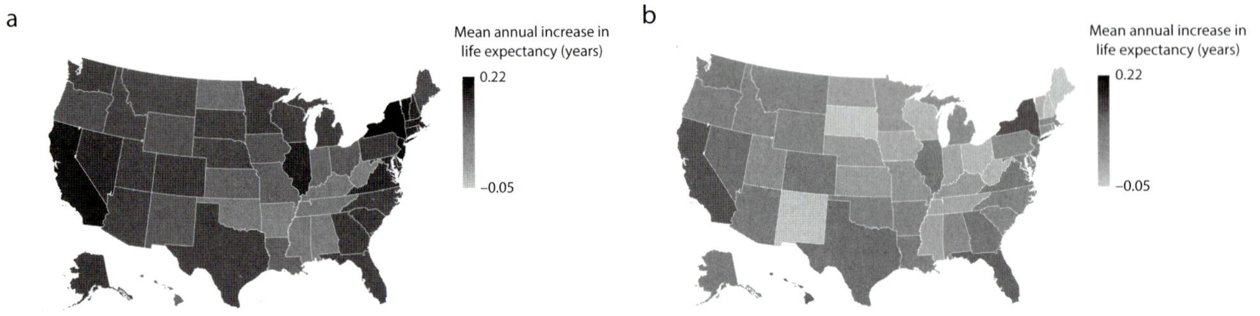

FIGURE 3— Mean Changes in Life Expectancy by State During (a) Phase 4, 1983–2009, and (b) Phase 5, 2010–2019: United States

Note. The maps depict mean changes in life expectancy per annum that states experienced over the years comprising phase 4 (1983–2009), when increases in US life expectancy slowed, and phase 5 (2010–2019), when US life expectancy stagnated.
Source. Author's calculations based on US Mortality Database.[11]

inflection points and slopes through statistical modeling (e.g., Joinpoint Regression Program). Finally, data from countries with relatively small populations can provide important insights but are sometimes less generalizable to large countries like the United States, where scalability and cross-cultural adaptability pose greater challenges.

Public Health Implications

The pervasiveness of the US health disadvantage, which involves dozens of diseases and causes of death and has lasted decades, suggests that the problem is larger and more enduring than any single health problem (e.g., drugs, firearms, obesity) and likely involves upstream, systemic factors capable of producing widespread effects on health.[1] Health is not the only domain in which the United States has lost ground to other countries, further indication that systemic obstacles and policy choices may have impeded socioeconomic progress on a more fundamental level. For example, despite its vast aggregate wealth, the United States has the highest income inequality (e.g., Gini coefficient), greatest concentration of wealth, and highest poverty rate in the Organisation for Economic Co-operation and Development.[25] Since 1995, 17 Organisation for Economic Co-operation and Development countries have surpassed the United States on the share of the population with a tertiary education.[25] In 2018, US students ranked 32nd in math performance at aged 15 years.[25] Such declines may reflect the rise of neoliberal policies, beginning in the 1970s, which were intentional about promoting entrepreneurial freedom and deregulation, redistributing wealth from the middle to the upper class, and curbing government's role in broadening access to education, health care, and human services.[26]

Social and economic stresses, resulting in part from such policies, may help explain the geographic variation and slower growth in life expectancy observed in certain states. Although Appalachia and the Deep South (i.e., South Central and South Atlantic divisions) typically rank lowest on life expectancy and other health statistics,[27] I found that the slowest growth in life expectancy occurred not only in South Central states but also in the Midwest. The Midwest accounted for more than half of US states that experienced a decline in life expectancy in 2010 to 2019. Other studies found that the increase in midlife mortality that followed 2010—much of it driven by drug overdoses, suicide, and liver disease—was disproportionately concentrated in the Industrial Midwest.[7,28,29] States in the Rust Belt and agricultural heartland endured the collapse of the manufacturing sector and the farm crisis, which claimed jobs and family farms, increased economic precarity, and potentially compromised health outcomes.[30,31] These states also underwent a political shift to more conservative policies on matters that affect health (e.g., Medicaid eligibility, tobacco taxes, social welfare).[32] Studies show that states that adopted more conservative policies were more likely to experience stagnant or decreasing life expectancy and higher mortality even after adjustment for confounding variables.[32]

Whether these factors are causally implicated in the US life expectancy disadvantage or the geographic variation observed here will require additional research using innovative study designs that can distinguish between mediators and confounding variables. A range of potential systemic explanations for the US health disadvantage should be considered. Structural racism, for example, produces deep health inequities among people of color but may also adversely affect the White population.[33] Investigators should also explore the contribution of diet, psychosocial factors, trauma, despair (particularly among young adults[34,35]), disruptions in family structure, economic hypersegregation of communities, political polarization, erosions in social cohesion and trust, and harmful technological influences (e.g., social media), among others.

Although these research priorities are important, the US health disadvantage continues to claim lives in real time. The crisis has broad implications, affecting not only mortality but also morbidity, with ripple effects on health care costs, workforce productivity, and the economy. The gravity of the situation may justify intervention even before definitive evidence becomes available. A prudent first step would be to examine policies that have enabled other countries to consistently outperform the United States for decades. AJPH

ABOUT THE AUTHOR

Steven H. Woolf is with the Center on Society and Health and the Department of Family Medicine and Population Health, Virginia Commonwealth University, Richmond.

CORRESPONDENCE

Correspondence should be sent to Steven H. Woolf, MD, MPH, Center on Society and Health, Virginia Commonwealth University School of Medicine, 830 East Main St, Suite 5035, Richmond, VA 23298-0212 (e-mail: steven.woolf@vcuhealth.org). Reprints can be ordered at http://www.ajph.org by clicking the "Reprints" link.

PUBLICATION INFORMATION

Full Citation: Woolf SH. Falling behind: the growing gap in life expectancy between the United States and other countries, 1933–2021. *Am J Public Health*. 2023;113(9):970–980.

Acceptance Date: March 28, 2023.

DOI: https://doi.org/10.2105/AJPH.2023.307310

ACKNOWLEDGMENTS

S. H. Woolf received partial funding from the National Center for Advancing Translational Sciences (grant UM1TR004360).

The author thanks Jong Hyung Lee, PhD, for his assistance with mapping.

CONFLICTS OF INTEREST

The author has no conflicts of interest to report.

HUMAN PARTICIPANT PROTECTION

The study did not involve human participants and was therefore exempt from institutional review under federal regulation 45 CFR 46.101(b; 4).

REFERENCES

1. Woolf SH, Aron LY, eds. *US Health in International Perspective: Shorter Lives, Poorer Health.* Washington, DC: National Academies Press; 2013.
2. Woolf SH, Masters RK, Aron LY. Effect of the COVID-19 pandemic in 2020 on life expectancy across populations in the USA and other high income countries: simulations of provisional mortality data. *BMJ*. 2021;373(1343):n1343. https://doi.org/10.1136/bmj.n1343
3. Islam N, Jdanov DA, Shkolnikov VM, et al. Effects of COVID-19 pandemic on life expectancy and premature mortality in 2020: time series analysis in 37 countries. *BMJ*. 2021;375:e066768. https://doi.org/10.1136/bmj-2021-066768
4. Arias E, Tejada-Vera B, Kochanek KD, Ahmad FB. *Provisional Life Expectancy Estimates for 2021.* Hyattsville, MD: National Center for Health Statistics; August 2022. Vital Statistics Rapid Release, no 23.
5. Crimmins EM, Preston SH, Cohen B, eds. *Explaining Divergent Levels of Longevity in High-Income Countries.* Washington, DC: National Academies Press; 2011.
6. Ho JY, Hendi AS. Recent trends in life expectancy across high income countries: retrospective observational study. *BMJ*. 2018;362:k2562. https://doi.org/10.1136/bmj.k2562
7. Becker T, Majmundar MK, Harris KM, eds. *High and Rising Mortality Rates Among Working-Age Adults.* Washington, DC: National Academies Press; 2021.
8. Ho JY. Causes of America's lagging life expectancy: an international comparative perspective. *J Gerontol B Psychol Sci Soc Sci.* 2022;77(suppl 2):S117–S126. https://doi.org/10.1093/geronb/gbab129
9. United Nations, Department of Economic and Social Affairs, Population Division. *World Population Prospects 2022.* Available at: https://population.un.org/wpp/Download/Standard/MostUsed. Accessed October 27, 2022.
10. Max Planck Institute for Demographic Research; University of California, Berkeley; French Institute for Demographic Studies. Human Mortality Database. Available at: www.mortality.org. Accessed October 29, 2022.
11. Barbieri M, Wilmoth J. US mortality database. Available at: https://usa.mortality.org. Accessed October 31, 2022.
12. United Nations, Department of Economic and Social Affairs, Population Division. *World Population Prospects 2022: Methodology of the United Nations Population Estimates and Projections.* Available at: https://population.un.org/wpp/Publications/Files/WPP2022_Methodology.pdf. Accessed November 11, 2022.
13. United Nations, Department of Economic and Social Affairs, Population Division. *World Population Prospects 2022: Data Sources.* Available at: https://population.un.org/wpp/Download/Files/4_Metadata/WPP2022_Data_Sources.pdf. Accessed November 11, 2022.
14. United Nations, Department of Economic and Social Affairs, Statistics Division. Methodology: standard country or area codes for statistical use (M49). Available at: https://unstats.un.org/unsd/methodology/m49. Accessed November 28, 2022.
15. World Bank. World Bank analytical classifications. Available at: http://databank.worldbank.org/data/download/site-content/OGHIST.xlsx. Accessed September 24, 2022.
16. World Bank. *World Development Report, 1978.* Washington, DC; 1978. Available at: http://documents.worldbank.org/curated/en/297241468339565863/World-development-report-1978. Accessed April 5, 2023.
17. Nations of the World. The continents of the world. Available at: https://www.nationsonline.org/oneworld/continents.htm. Accessed November 11, 2022.
18. US Census Bureau. Census regions and divisions of the United States. Available at: https://www2.census.gov/geo/pdfs/maps-data/maps/reference/us_regdiv.pdf. Accessed November 11, 2022.
19. Beckfield J, Bambra C. Shorter lives in stingier states: social policy shortcomings help explain the US mortality disadvantage. *Soc Sci Med.* 2016;171:30–38. https://doi.org/10.1016/j.socscimed.2016.10.017
20. Reynolds MM, Avendano M. Social policy expenditures and life expectancy in high-income countries. *Am J Prev Med.* 2018;54(1):72–79. https://doi.org/10.1016/j.amepre.2017.09.001
21. Case A, Deaton A. Mortality and morbidity in the 21st century. *Brookings Pap Econ Act.* 2017;2017(1):397–476. https://doi.org/10.1353/eca.2017.0005
22. Woolf SH, Chapman DA, Buchanich JM, Bobby KJ, Zimmerman EB, Blackburn SM. Changes in midlife death rates across racial and ethnic groups in the United States: systematic analysis of vital statistics. *BMJ*. 2018;362:k3096. https://doi.org/10.1136/bmj.k3096
23. Schöley J, Aburto JM, Kashnitsky I, et al. Life expectancy changes since COVID-19. *Nat Hum Behav.* 2022;6(12):1649–1659. https://doi.org/10.1038/s41562-022-01450-3
24. Wilmoth JR, Andreev K, Jdanov D, et al. Methods protocol for the Human Mortality Database. May 31, 2007. Available at: https://v5.mortality.org/Public/Docs/MethodsProtocol.pdf. Accessed November 28, 2022.
25. Organisation for Economic Cooperation and Development. OECD data. Available at: https://data.oecd.org. Accessed October 9, 2022.
26. Harvey D. *A Brief History of Neoliberalism.* New York, NY: Oxford University Press; 2005.
27. United Health Foundation. America's health rankings, 2019. Available at: https://www.americashealthrankings.org/learn/reports/2019-annual-report. Accessed November 28, 2022.
28. Woolf SH, Schoomaker H. Life expectancy and mortality rates in the United States, 1959–2017. *JAMA.* 2019;322(20):1996–2016. https://doi.org/10.1001/jama.2019.16932
29. Stein EM, Gennuso KP, Ugboaja DC, Remington PL. The epidemic of despair among White

Americans: trends in the leading causes of premature death, 1999–2015. *Am J Public Health.* 2017;107(10):1541–1547. https://doi.org/10.2105/AJPH.2017.303941

30. Barnett BJ. The US farm financial crisis of the 1980s. *Agric Hist.* 2000;74(2):366–380. https://doi.org/10.1215/00021482-74.2.366
31. Venkataramani AS, Bair EF, O'Brien RL, Tsai AC. Association between automotive assembly plant closures and opioid overdose mortality in the United States: a difference-in-differences analysis. *JAMA Intern Med.* 2020;180(2):254–262. https://doi.org/10.1001/jamainternmed.2019.5686
32. Montez JK, Mehri N, Monnat SM, et al. US state policy contexts and mortality of working-age adults. *PLoS One.* 2022;17(10):e0275466. https://doi.org/10.1371/journal.pone.0275466
33. Malat J, Mayorga-Gallo S, Williams DR. The effects of Whiteness on the health of Whites in the USA. *Soc Sci Med.* 2018;199:148–156. https://doi.org/10.1016/j.socscimed.2017.06.034
34. Gaydosh L, Hummer RA, Hargrove TW, et al. The depths of despair among US adults entering midlife. *Am J Public Health.* 2019;109(5):774–780. https://doi.org/10.2105/AJPH.2019.305002
35. Shanahan L, Hill SN, Gaydosh LM, et al. Does despair really kill? A roadmap for an evidence-based answer. *Am J Public Health.* 2019;109(6):854–858. https://doi.org/10.2105/AJPH.2019.305016

Ambient Temperature and Emergency Hospital Admissions in People Experiencing Homelessness: London, United Kingdom, 2011–2019

Shakoor Hajat, PhD, MSc, Christophe E. Sarran, PhD, MPhys, Mariya Bezgrebelna, MA, and Sean A. Kidd, PhD, CPsych

Objectives. To assess the impacts of ambient temperature on hospitalizations of people experiencing homelessness.

Methods. We used daily time-series regression analysis employing distributed lag nonlinear models of 148 177 emergency inpatient admissions with "no fixed abode" and 20 804 admissions with a diagnosis of homelessness in London, United Kingdom, in 2011 through 2019.

Results. There was a significantly increased risk of hospitalization associated with high temperature; at 25°C versus the minimum morbidity temperature (MMT), relative risks were 1.359 (95% confidence interval [CI] = 1.216, 1.580) and 1.351 (95% CI = 1.039, 1.757) for admissions with "no fixed abode" and admissions with a homelessness diagnosis, respectively. Between 14.5% and 18.9% of admissions were attributable to temperatures above the MMT. No significant associations were observed with cold.

Conclusions. There is an elevated risk of hospitalization associated with even moderately high temperatures in individuals experiencing homelessness. Risks are larger than those reported in the general population.

Public Health Implications. Greater emphasis should be placed on addressing homeless vulnerabilities during hot weather rather than cold. Activation thresholds for interventions such as the Severe Weather Emergency Protocol (SWEP) could be better aligned with health risks. Given elevated risks at even moderate temperatures, our findings support prioritization of prevention-oriented measures, rather than crisis response, to address homelessness. (*Am J Public Health*. 2023;113(9): 981–984. https://doi.org/10.2105/AJPH.2023.307351)

AJPH September 2023, Vol 113, No. 9

The impacts of climate change and extreme weather on the health of people who lack adequate shelter have received little attention.[1] Homeless populations have specific health and social vulnerabilities that heighten risk of illness and death during severe weather. Climate change means that rough sleepers are exposed not only to severe winter weather but also increasingly higher ambient temperatures, particularly in heavily urbanized cities such as London, United Kingdom, where heat stress can be amplified because of the Urban Heat Island.[2] Heat impacts are also intensified by risk factors common in rough sleepers and those with insecure housing, such as the presence of underlying physical and mental health conditions, drug and alcohol dependencies, reduced access to air-conditioned environments and drinking water, and social isolation.[3]

As the United Kingdom continues to experience greater climate extremes, there is an urgent need to assess the health impacts of ambient heat and cold exposure in homeless populations. People experiencing homelessness face barriers accessing primary health care, leading to higher rates of attendance at emergency departments.

Health care costs for people experiencing homelessness are 8 times greater than for the general population and hospital stays are 3 times longer,[4] so evidence-informed interventions can help ease burdens on the National Health Service (NHS).

We aimed to characterize the impacts of ambient temperature on emergency hospital admissions by people experiencing homelessness in Greater London, which hosts about 30% of the country's homeless population. Given the heightened exposures and vulnerabilities of the homeless population, we hypothesized that adverse impacts occur at even moderate temperatures.

METHODS

We collected daily counts of emergency hospital inpatient admissions between 2011 and 2019 recorded on the Hospital Episode Statistics database by NHS Digital. We identified contacts by individuals experiencing homelessness using 2 fields: (1) all-cause admissions, where residential address was recorded as "no fixed abode" (pseudo postal district code ZZ99); (2) where a primary or secondary diagnosis of homelessness was recorded (*International Classification of Diseases, 10th Revision* [ICD-10], code Z59.0). Days with admission counts of 5 or fewer were not available to preserve patient anonymity and so were set to missing. We obtained daily maximum and minimum temperature data from the Met Office using the HadUK-Grid data set, which interpolates observations from land-surface monitoring stations onto a uniform 1-km grid.[5] From this, we created composite temperature series representing the whole of London by averaging values from contributing grid cells.

We used Quasi–Poisson time-series regression to assess short-term associations between daily temperature (maximum or minimum) and hospital counts, adjusting for trends and underlying seasonal patterns (unrelated to temperature) using natural cubic splines with 7 degrees of freedom per year and indicator terms for day of week.[6] The trend and seasonal controls ensure that temporal changes in the size of the population and other confounding factors that change slowly over time are inherently controlled for. We used distributed lag nonlinear models (DLNMs) employing cross-basis functions to flexibly model nonlinear and delayed effects of temperature.[7] This framework allows quantification of risk at different values of the nonlinear temperature or lag distribution, as well as the summed effect. The model is summarized:

$$\text{(1)}\quad \text{Log}[E(Y_i)] = \alpha + \beta_1 T_{i,j} + \beta_2 \text{ncs}(\text{time}_i,\ \text{df} = 7/\text{year}) + \beta_3(\text{dow}_i)$$

where $E[Y_i]$ is expected admissions on day i, $T_{i,j}$ is the cross-basis matrix of temperature and lag j up to 21 days, ncs = natural cubic spline functions, and dow = day-of-week indicator. Although we considered lagged effects up to 21 days, heat impacts in particular are likely to be more immediate and so we also considered shorter lag structures in the DLNMs, but results were robust to such specifications.

For each field, we identified the minimum morbidity temperature (MMT) at which risk of admission is lowest, and estimated the relative risk (RR) of admission at selected temperatures compared with the MMT. We also quantified attributable fractions of temperatures above the MMT.

RESULTS

During 2011 to 2019, there was a minimum of 148 177 emergency inpatient admissions in London categorized as "no fixed abode" and 20 804 where the primary or secondary diagnosis was recorded as homelessness. Figure A (available as a supplement to the online version of this article at http://www.ajph.org) shows daily counts of admissions with "no fixed abode," which generally exhibits yearly summertime peaks. The trend of increasing admissions mirrors general increases in hospitalization numbers,[8] although the number of rough sleepers in London is also known to have increased during this period.[9] The average daily counts for the "no fixed abode" and homelessness diagnosis variables were 45.9 and 10.2, respectively.

Figure 1 shows the seasonally adjusted relationship between daily maximum temperature and the relative risk of admission for those with "no fixed abode." The figure shows increased risk of admission associated with high temperature. Compared with a MMT of 6°C, a value of 25°C (approximately the 93rd percentile) was associated with an RR of 1.359 (95% confidence interval [CI] = 1.216, 1.580). Temperatures above the MMT accounted for 18.9% of all admissions. We observed a similar relationship with the homelessness diagnosis outcome (not shown), with an RR of 1.351 (95% CI = 1.039, 1.757) at 25°C compared with a MMT of 9°C, and temperatures above the MMT accounting for 14.5% of admissions. Cold effects were not statistically significant, including when minimum temperature was the exposure.

DISCUSSION

Our results show that ambient heat is an important risk factor for emergency

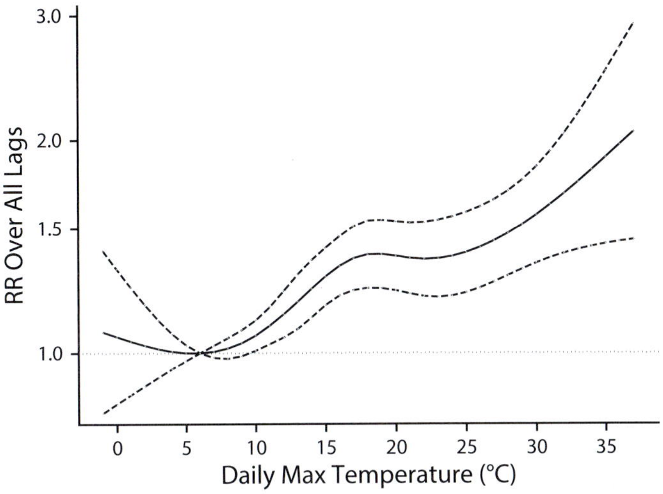

FIGURE 1— Seasonally Adjusted Relationship Between Daily Maximum Temperature (°C) and Relative Risk (RR) of Emergency Hospital Admissions Classified as "No Fixed Abode": London, United Kingdom, 2011–2019

Note. The dashed lines indicate 95% confidence intervals.

hospital admissions among people experiencing homelessness. Risks are greater than those recently reported for the general population of England using a similar methodology,[10] reflecting heightened vulnerabilities for individuals experiencing homelessness. Likewise, US studies have shown particularly high odds of emergency department visits and deaths in homeless groups during hot weather.[11,12] We observed no significantly raised risk associated with low temperatures, which agrees with evidence from emergency department attendances in North England.[13] This may reflect better risk perception and preventative action taken by individuals experiencing homelessness and by homeless organizations during cold weather.

Admissions by individuals experiencing homelessness are likely to be underreported because a homelessness diagnosis is only recorded if a clinician considers it clinically relevant. Our reliance on this as a diagnosis had evident power limitations, so we also considered "no fixed abode" as an alternative indicator of homelessness, which is more numerous but less specific because it also captures people not experiencing homelessness who may wish to conceal their real address. The 2 outcomes, however, yielded very similar results. Days with 0 to 5 admission counts were unavailable, so their exclusion may have introduced bias; however, this applied to only 1.8% of days for "no fixed abode," and results were largely unchanged when these days were assigned a nominal count of 3 for both outcomes in sensitivity analysis. Although we observed little cold effect, future research could consider potential impacts of other wintry weather such as snowfall and rainfall.

PUBLIC HEALTH IMPLICATIONS

Our study indicates that more emphasis should be placed on addressing homeless vulnerabilities during hot weather rather than cold. In England, the main recognition of climate vulnerabilities in the homeless population is through the Severe Weather Emergency Protocol (SWEP), which supports local authorities to issue an emergency response during extreme weather.[14] Traditionally focused on cold weather, heat wave guidance is also now incorporated into SWEP, although our results indicate that the summertime SWEP activation threshold of 25°C maximum temperature is already associated with a 35% increased risk of hospitalization. Adverse health impacts occur at even moderate temperatures, and the high estimated heat-attributable fractions are mostly from moderate temperature days rather than the infrequent extreme temperature days when SWEP operates. Although SWEP is primarily an emergency response designed to provide overnight shelter for rough sleepers rather than engagement with health services, our results suggest that if it seeks to reach individuals experiencing homelessness before their health is compromised, existing activation thresholds may need to be revised. The elevated health risks observed in our study at even moderate temperatures support prioritization of prevention-oriented measures, rather than crisis response, to address homelessness. AJPH

ABOUT THE AUTHORS

Shakoor Hajat is with the London School of Hygiene & Tropical Medicine, London, UK. Christophe E. Sarran is with the Met Office, Exeter, UK. Mariya Bezgrebelna is with the Department of Psychology, York University, Toronto, Ontario, Canada. Sean A. Kidd is with the Centre for Addiction and Mental Health and the University of Toronto Department of Psychiatry, Toronto.

CORRESPONDENCE

Correspondence should be sent to Professor Shakoor Hajat, Centre on Climate Change and Planetary Health, Department of Public Health, Environments and Society, 15-17 Tavistock Place, London WC1H 9SH, UK (e-mail: shakoor.hajat@lshtm.ac.uk). Reprints can be ordered at http://www.ajph.org by clicking the "Reprints" link.

PUBLICATION INFORMATION

Full Citation: Hajat S, Sarran CE, Bezgrebelna M, Kidd SA. Ambient temperature and emergency hospital admissions in people experiencing homelessness: London, United Kingdom, 2011–2019. *Am J Public Health*. 2023;113(9): 981–984.

Acceptance Date: May 20, 2023.

DOI: https://doi.org/10.2105/AJPH.2023.307351

CONTRIBUTORS

S. Hajat performed study conceptualization, statistical analyses, and article writing. C. E Sarran performed data processing, article review, and feedback. M. Bezgrebelna performed article review and feedback. S. A. Kidd performed article review and feedback. All authors approved the final draft of the article.

ACKNOWLEDGMENTS

This study was partly funded by the National Institute for Health and Care Research (NIHR) Health Protection Research Unit in Environmental Change and Health (NIHR200909), a partnership between the London School of Hygiene & Tropical Medicine, the UK Health Security Agency, University College London, and the Met Office.

Note. The views expressed are those of the authors and not necessarily those of the NIHR, UK Health Security Agency, or the Department of Health and Social Care.

CONFLICTS OF INTEREST

The authors have no conflicts of interest to report.

HUMAN PARTICIPANT PROTECTION

This study did not involve human participants.

REFERENCES

1. Kidd SA, Hajat S, Bezgrebelna M, McKenzie K. The climate change–homelessness nexus. *Lancet*. 2021;397(10286):1693–1694. https://doi.org/10.1016/S0140-6736(21)00834-5
2. Ramin B, Svoboda T. Health of the homeless and climate change. *J Urban Health*. 2009;86(4):654–664. https://doi.org/10.1007/s11524-009-9354-7
3. Hajat S, O'Connor M, Kosatsky T. Health effects of hot weather: from awareness of risk factors to effective health protection. *Lancet*. 2010; 375(9717):856–863. https://doi.org/10.1016/S0140-6736(09)61711-6
4. Thomas B. *Homelessness Kills: An Analysis of the Mortality of Homeless People in Early Twenty-First Century England*. London, UK: University of Sheffield and Crisis; 2012.
5. HadUK-Grid. Gridded climate observations for the UK. Met Office. Available at: https://www.metoffice.gov.uk/research/climate/maps-and-data/data/haduk-grid/haduk-grid. Accessed December 1, 2022.
6. Bhaskaran K, Gasparrini A, Hajat S, Smeeth L, Armstrong B. Time series regression studies in environmental epidemiology. *Int J Epidemiol*. 2013;42(4):1187–1195. https://doi.org/10.1093/ije/dyt092
7. Armstrong B. Models for the relationship between ambient temperature and daily mortality. *Epidemiology*. 2006;17(6):624–631. https://doi.org/10.1097/01.ede.0000239732.50999.8f
8. NHS England. A&E attendances and emergency admissions 2020. Available at: https://www.england.nhs.uk/statistics/statistical-work-areas/ae-waiting-times-and-activity. Accessed May 3, 2023.
9. Ministry of Housing, Communities and Local Government. Rough sleeping snapshot in England: autumn 2019. 2020. Available at: https://www.gov.uk/government/statistics/rough-sleeping-snapshot-in-england-autumn-2019/rough-sleeping-snapshot-in-england-autumn-2019#annex-regional-maps. Accessed May 3, 2023.
10. Rizmie D, de Preux L, Miraldo M, Atun R. Impact of extreme temperatures on emergency hospital admissions by age and socio-economic deprivation in England. *Soc Sci Med*. 2022;308:115193. https://doi.org/10.1016/j.socscimed.2022.115193
11. Schwarz L, Castillo EM, Chan TC, et al. Heat waves and emergency department visits among the homeless, San Diego, 2012–2019. *Am J Public Health*. 2022;112(1):98–106. https://doi.org/10.2105/AJPH.2021.306557
12. Harlan SL, Declet-Barreto JH, Stefanov WL, Petitti DB. Neighborhood effects on heat deaths: social and environmental predictors of vulnerability in Maricopa County, Arizona. *Environ Health Perspect*. 2013;121(2):197–204. https://doi.org/10.1289/ehp.1104625
13. Brown AJ, Goodacre SW, Cross S. Do emergency department attendances by homeless people increase in cold weather? *Emerg Med J*. 2010;27(7): 526–529. https://doi.org/10.1136/emj.2009.076679
14. Severe Weather Emergency Protocol. Homeless Link. Available at: https://homelesslink-1b54.kxcdn.com/media/documents/Severe_Weather_Emergency_Protocol_FAQs_February_2020_9KRmXPP.pdf. Accessed August 12, 2022.

Lessons Ignored: Children and Pandemics

Cynthia Connolly, RN, PhD, and Janet Golden, PhD

Children became sick and died during pandemics roughly 100 years apart, but they are rarely the central focus of historical scholarship. Because children were not the largest group of victims in the 1918 pandemic or in the COVID-19 pandemic and because of their lack of political capital, their needs received little attention. Both pandemics exposed the many holes in the nation's health and welfare infrastructure. We examine responses to children's needs in Philadelphia, Pennsylvania, during the peak pandemic year of 1918 and then show how this legacy of the lack of any child policy infrastructure left the city underresourced during the COVID-19 pandemic. (*Am J Public Health*. 2023;113(9):985–990. https://doi.org/10.2105/AJPH.2023.307334)

The 2020 COVID-19 pandemic arrived in a far different world than the so-called Spanish influenza pandemic more than a century earlier. People and governments in both eras attempted to address the challenges of a deadly outbreak. Despite the cataclysmic impact on Americans in each era, neither the 1918 pandemic nor apparently the COVID-19 pandemic transformed American traditions of reliance on short-term, targeted, and means-tested social programs to support children. Because children were not the largest group of victims in the 1918 pandemic or in the COVID-19 pandemic and because of their lack of political influence, their needs received little attention. This was true even as their experiences in both pandemics exposed the many holes in the nation's health and welfare infrastructure.

The plight of children during pandemics provokes immediate sympathy and short-term interventions but no permanent programs aimed at improving their well-being. We illustrate this argument by examining responses to children's needs in Philadelphia, Pennsylvania, during the peak pandemic year of 1918 and then by showing how the lack of any federal child policy infrastructure left the city underresourced during the COVID-19 pandemic.

The 1918 influenza pandemic hit Philadelphia in September, and case rates climbed in the weeks that followed. The Department of Public Health and Charities closed schools, churches, theaters, and other places of public assembly and told people to stay home from work if they became sick. Ten temporary hospitals opened to provide care, including some in clubs and churches. Voluntary organizations helped transport doctors and nurses, and off-duty police, firefighters, and teachers stepped up to deliver food and other forms of assistance.

With physicians and nurses absent on World War I military service, medical students from the city's closed medical colleges attended to patients as did nursing students, volunteers from women's groups, and members of religious organizations. Even volunteer gravediggers did their part as the city struggled to deal with the growing numbers of bodies and insufficient space in the city morgue. The pandemic peaked and ebbed rapidly, leaving thousands of Philadelphians dead, in part as a result of a mass public gathering for a World War I Liberty Loan parade.[1]

CHILDREN AND THE 1918 INFLUENZA PANDEMIC IN PHILADELPHIA

The greatest number of deaths occurred among individuals 20 to 40 years of age, but Philadelphia's infants and children suffered as well (Figure 1). The city's infant mortality rate, the fourth highest in the nation, remained stubbornly high through the outbreak. Before the pandemic hit, 1918 had been a difficult year for the city's youngest citizens. An extra-cold winter combined with a coal shortage meant that the most vulnerable families, such as those in the tenement districts, struggled to keep warm, whereas

AJPH September 2023, Vol 113, No. 9

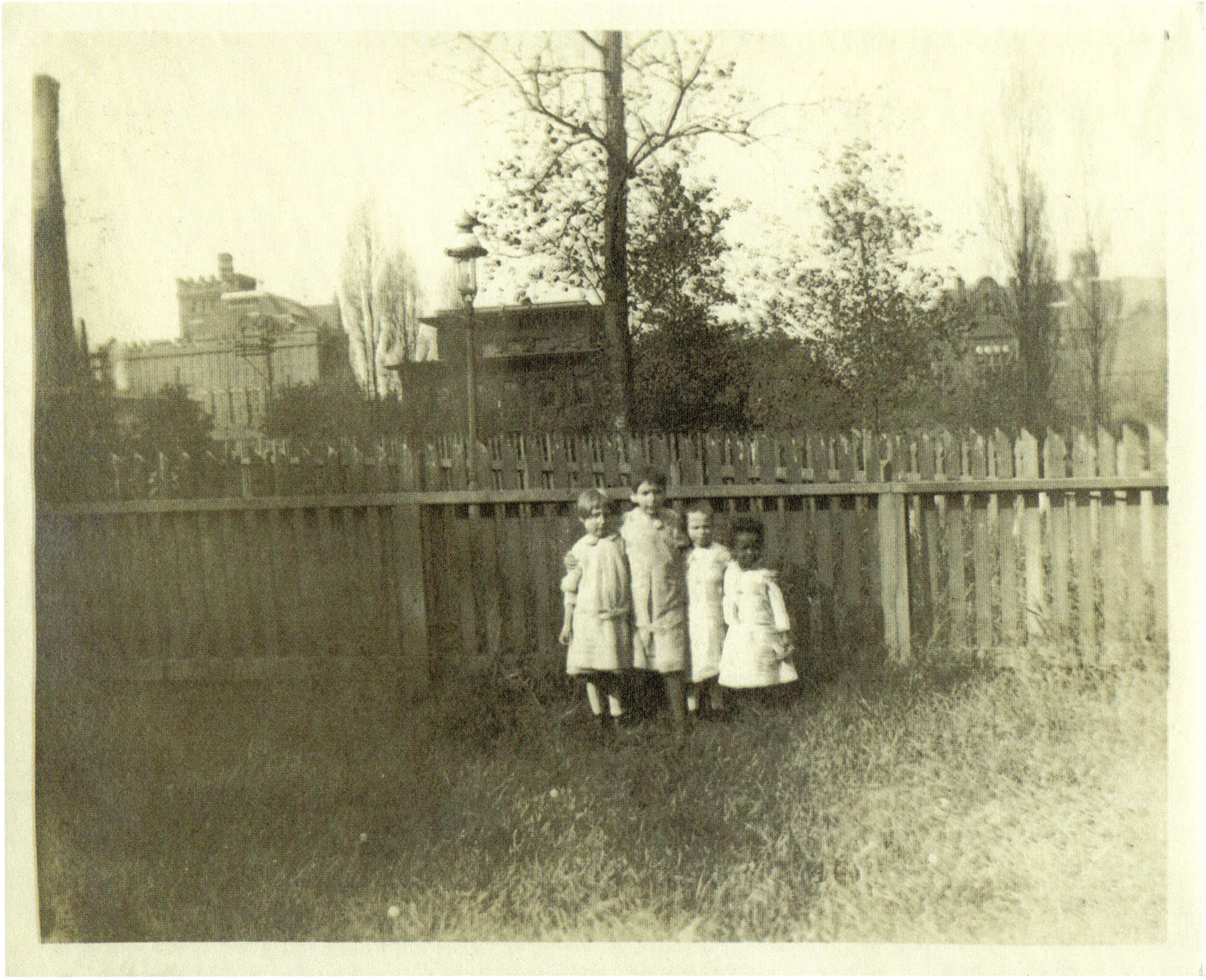

FIGURE 1— Four Philadelphia Children, September 28, 1918

Source. Alumni Association of the Philadelphia General Hospital School of Nursing Image Collection, Barbara Bates Center for the Study of the History of Nursing, School of Nursing, University of Pennsylvania. Printed with permission.

high coal prices left parents with less money to purchase food and milk for their children. Even middle-class families struggled to make ends meet. In the unusually hot summer that followed, with temperatures as high as 106 degrees, food and milk quickly spoiled, heightening children's risk for life-threatening dehydration and infectious diarrheal diseases.[2]

The flu added an unprecedented level of anxiety to parents who feared for their children. As an example of the chaos and breakdown of order wrought by the flu, one Philadelphia newspaper article reported that a group of mothers in a working-class neighborhood surrounded a physician's car demanding that he visit their ill children. In the next few hours, the doctor made house calls to 57 extremely ill children.[3]

In March 1919, physician Harriet L. Hartley, chief of the Philadelphia Health Department's Bureau of Child Hygiene, alerted her colleagues that the pandemic's severe consequences for the city's infants and young children did not come into focus until the pandemic was over. It was only then that she and others were able to drill deeper into pandemic-related data. Hartley reminded her colleagues that at the beginning of the pandemic even some experts believed that infants and young children were "escaping" the flu. However, of the more than 12 000 recorded deaths from flu-related causes in fall 1918, she noted that almost 2000 occurred among children younger than 5 years. The 1918 infant mortality rate in Philadelphia increased by 16% over

AJPH September 2023, Vol 113, No. 9

the rate in 1917, with most of the deaths occurring during the pandemic.[4]

Hartley also documented that many children who did not contract the flu themselves suffered because of its impact on their households. With schools closed for weeks, thousands of Philadelphia youngsters played in the streets at heightened risk for accidents and saw dead bodies left outside to be taken to the overwhelmed city morgue. Thousands of orphaned Philadelphia children and those whose parents were in the hospital or sick at home languished, becoming malnourished, dehydrated, or ill from lack of monitoring.[5]

As the numbers of sick and dying adults rose, public health officials diverted resources budgeted for Philadelphia's children to pandemic mitigation. They redirected nurses employed by the Division of Child Hygiene of the Philadelphia Health Department to care for hospitalized adults.[6] In response to the lack of trained nursing staff and pediatric beds, the city turned to the Catholic church. Nuns quickly reconfigured a school into an emergency pediatric hospital for the city's poorest, identified as the "colored people, the Italians, the others of God's poor."[7]

Fortunately, children suffering from the flu who made it to the hospital were overwhelmingly likely to survive.[8] However, finding a place to discharge children whose parents remained sick or who had died posed a problem. The Hospital of the University of Pennsylvania's Ward G, for example, admitted a number of children in late 1918 as a result of the flu or the life-threatening pneumonia that sometimes accompanied it. As noted by the children's worker hired by the Ward G Women's Auxiliary, hospital discharges posed challenges because of limited places to send recovering children and difficulty coordinating services among agencies. One patient admitted in the fall proved ready to go home by December 1918. The worker noted that the patient had improved enough from the flu and pneumonia that his "mind had cleared and his bodily strength returned." However, he could not go home because his mother was still too weak from her case of the flu.

Just as orphanages served "half-orphans" who could not be cared for at home, Ward G served as a waystation for those in similar circumstances.[9] In January 1919, the children's worker described the case of Mary, a child admitted to the ward with flu whose only parent, her father, was still hospitalized with flu next door at the municipal Philadelphia General Hospital. Mary had no one to care for her and was bound for foster care or an orphanage. Similarly, 4-year-old Adam's mother and infant brother had died of flu; he survived. With his father unable to work or care for him because of what had been diagnosed as epilepsy, Adam was transferred to the Children's Seashore House in Atlantic City, New Jersey.

The Ward G notes show the sympathy of the children's worker for the children's plight and at times her harsh judgments of the conditions in which immigrant and African American parents reared their children. As the worker noted, one father was able and willing to pay and anxious to learn how to care for his children. However, she reported that "the sanitary conditions are bad at this home." Nowhere does she address the poverty that resulted in bad hygiene and poor nutrition and their consequences.[10]

Caring for children outside of hospitals represented an even greater and more urgent challenge. The Catholic volunteers and nuns who provided aid to families in their homes identified horrific conditions. Children, both well and sick, huddled next to ill parents in homes with no heat, hot water, or food. In one household, they found that a dead child had lain for days next to sick parents and siblings.[11] The progressive journal *The Survey* published an anecdote of a particularly upsetting Philadelphia case. Health visitors to a home found the husband dead and discovered that his wife, who had birthed twins a week earlier, had had only one apple to eat since then.[12]

There was no shortage of voluntary organizations trying to compensate for the lack of governmental initiatives. The Emergency Service of the Pennsylvania Council of the National Defense in the Influenza Crisis (created within weeks of the October 1918 outbreak), settlement houses, and the local Red Cross chapter all attempted to bring some semblance of order to the pandemic response and grappled with how best to help children and families affected by the flu.[13] The Philadelphia Society for Organizing Charity summarized the problem as it found itself overwhelmed by the need to assist "hundreds of fatherless and motherless children" in the wake of the pandemic.[14] Another leading private charity, the Children's Aid Society, lamented the many ways that the flu had "complicate[d] and increase[d]" the organization's work.

Even as its staff was decimated by the flu, the Children's Aid Society managed to arrange emergency or temporary care for many children whose parents were sick or had died. Months later the society's officials believed that they still had not felt the full effect of the pandemic, noting that "every few days children are brought to us for care, because they are homeless as a result of the loss of one and sometimes both parents on account of the pandemic." They expected this disruption to last well into 1920.[15]

The flu overwhelmed Philadelphia's visiting nurse societies, the backbone of in-home health care in the city. According to the annual report of the Visiting Nurse Society of Philadelphia, many of the society's worst cases involved children who were caring for sick parents and siblings in homes without water, heat, and food. In addition to the actual care patients required, nurses struggled to meet other needs. They sought out family members or neighbors to care for the sick in their homes and placements for children whose parents were dead or too sick to care for them.[16] Visiting nurses documented many situations such as that of a 16-year-old boy who, after both parents died from the flu in quick succession, worried that he and his five younger siblings would be separated from one another.[17]

Despite the massive loss of life, World War I and the armistice that followed overshadowed the pandemic in public memory. Cities and towns erected war memorials but created no monuments to those who fought and sometimes died saving lives during the pandemic. The war stimulated creation of the modern American military but did not fundamentally alter the nation's public health and social welfare infrastructure. Some new social safety net programs promoting the well-being of children did emerge in the years that followed, including the Sheppard-Towner Maternity and Infancy Protection Act of 1921, which ended in 1929. This act funded state health promotion and education initiatives. Title V of the Social Security Act of 1935 provided means-tested financial support to the poorest families in many, but not all, states.[18] Another war, World War II, necessitated the Emergency Maternity and Infant Care Act. This program, which ran from 1943 to 1949, served the families of men in the lowest four pay grades, comprising 87% of all enlisted men.[19]

Even in the postwar economic and baby boom era, the federal government failed to secure the well-being of all of the nation's children. Medicaid, enacted in 1965, provided medical care for episodic illness to the nation's poorest children. Layered on top of previous programs, Medicaid continued the long-standing tradition of relying on a complicated and nonintegrated patchwork of programs, most of which were short term or means tested and often failed to reach minority households. Moreover, it did not mandate coverage for preventive screening and other health promotion initiatives. Congress attempted to address this issue in 1967, when it amended Medicaid to create the Early Periodic Screening, Diagnosis, and Treatment Act, which required states to provide childhood screening for developmental and other disorders as well as outreach regarding eligible services to the families covered by the program.[20]

NEW PANDEMIC: OLD STORY

As did other cities around the nation, Philadelphia confronted the COVID-19 crisis in an ad hoc fashion. The city established food distribution sites, and voluntary organizations and religious congregations also responded. With schools closed, the city's school district quickly established online programs, an effort that would ultimately yield diminished learning and great emotional distress relative to traditional in-school education. The school district distributed almost 8 million meals to children during the early part of the pandemic.[21]

Evidence emerged during the first pandemic year that although COVID-19 infections proved less deadly among children than adults, children were not immune. As early as November 2020, epidemiological data verified anecdotal reports that the overall risk of severe disease requiring hospitalization was low among children and adolescents. However, infection was more common and more severe among Black, Hispanic, and Asian adolescent patients and all youngsters with comorbidities.[22] Fortunately, Philadelphia reported no COVID-19 pediatric deaths, but the city did note increases in suicide, depression, and anxiety. Compounding the problem, schools and child-care centers lost staff members, and public health efforts to vaccinate children against COVID-19 and childhood diseases did not reach sufficient numbers of young people.[23]

Nationally as well as locally, adult deaths in the pandemic deprived children of parents, grandparents, and other relatives and friends. According to the Centers for Disease Control and Prevention (CDC), "from April 1, 2020 through June 30, 2021, data suggest that more than 140,000 children under age 18 in the United States lost a parent, custodial grandparent, or grandparent caregiver who provided the child's home and basic needs, including love, security, and daily care." Racial disparities characterized both the direct COVID-19 threat to children's health and the likelihood of losing a primary caregiver. Sixty-five percent of children who lost a primary caregiver were members of racial or ethnic minority groups. The CDC reported that "the highest burden of death fell on children living along the U.S.-Mexico border, in the South, and in tribal areas."[24]

In 2020 as in 1918, the fear of death was ever present. Children suffered emotionally as they watched the world around them, with their fears perhaps becoming even more vivid because of their exposure to so many types of media that did not exist in 1918. An article in the *Philadelphia Inquirer* in April 2020 told of a 9-year-old girl who "curled into a ball and sobbed for her dad, worried that he'd get the coronavirus while doing his job delivering prescription medications."[25]

Mass casualty events such as the COVID-19 pandemic that reached Philadelphia in 2020 leave their mark on survivors, whether they lost loved ones or experienced the trauma that grew from what they witnessed and feared. Pediatric and public health experts are now arguing for COVID-19 life course studies. Part of their rationale comes from an awareness of the fact that the social disruption and loss caused by the 1918 pandemic lingered for decades. Children born during that time were more likely to struggle with health-related issues throughout their lifetimes.[26] Just as Hartley and others observed in Philadelphia in 1919, subsequent research after the 1918 pandemic revealed that prematurity and infant death increased nationally. The full effects of the COVID-19 virus, particularly on children, may not be fully apparent for years or even decades.[27]

The 2021 American Rescue Plan Act, enacted under President Joseph R. Biden, dramatically reduced the child poverty rate while expanding access to food assistance and Medicaid. In Philadelphia, it enabled more than 26 000 children to receive medical care because of Medicaid expansion, provided additional funds to more than 169 000 families through the Child Care Tax Credit portion of the act, and supported food assistance to more than 172 000 families through expansion of the Supplemental Nutritional Assistance Program.[28]

Thus far, the COVID-19 pandemic has not resulted in permanent new programs designed to ensure the well-being of children despite all of the evidence of their needs. The fear that aid to children promotes and sustains a culture of dependency and undermines parents' work ethic—a long-standing belief that has shaped past social welfare programs—seems impervious to change. The recent effort to extend the Child Care Tax Credit, which dramatically reduced the child poverty rate, failed to become permanent. In an echo of the past, opponents voiced opposition to its costs and argued that providing cash to families would lead some parents to behave irresponsibly or use the funds to purchase drugs. New child and family support policies, opponents of making the Child Care Tax Credit permanent argued, needed both a parental work requirement and an income cap just as they had in the past.

Pandemics create immediate demands and require a rapid response. They stimulate both government bodies and private organizations to deliver direct services and deploy resources quickly to minimize morbidity and mortality. Yet, in the United States they have not left a legacy that addresses the need for robust and effective programs for children and families. Filling the gaps in health and social welfare that become visible in pandemics, past and present, has never stimulated enough political energy to make children a societal priority. The response to the 1918 pandemic did not become the foundation for a stable and robust system of health and social support in the 20th century. Thus far, the COVID-19 pandemic has not done so either. Perhaps the next pandemic will finally convey the importance of making child well-being a national priority. AJPH

ABOUT THE AUTHORS

Cynthia Connolly is with the Barbara Bates Center for the Study of the History of Nursing, University of Pennsylvania School of Nursing, Philadelphia. Janet Golden (retired) was formerly with the Department of History, Rutgers University–Camden, Camden, NJ.

CORRESPONDENCE

Correspondence should be sent to Cynthia Connolly, RN, PhD, University of Pennsylvania School of Nursing, 2017 Claire M. Fagin Hall, 418 Curie Blvd, Philadelphia, PA 19104-6020 (e-mail: cac1@nursing.upenn.edu). Reprints can be ordered at http://www.ajph.org by clicking the "Reprints" link.

PUBLICATION INFORMATION

Full Citation: Connolly C, Golden J. Lessons ignored: children and pandemics. *Am J Public Health*. 2023;113(9):985–990.

Acceptance Date: May 9, 2023.

DOI: https://doi.org/10.2105/AJPH.2023.307334

CONTRIBUTORS

The authors contributed equally to the research for and writing of this article.

CONFLICTS OF INTEREST

The authors have no conflicts of interest to disclose.

ENDNOTES

1. James E. Higgins, "A Lost History: Writing the Influenza Epidemic in Pennsylvania, 1918–1922," *Pennsylvania History* 85, no. 3 (2018): 394–405; Jeffrey S. Anderson, "'When We Have a Few More Epidemics the City Officials Will Awake': Philadelphia and the Influenza Epidemic of 1918–1919," *The Maryland Historian* 27, no. 1/2 (1996): 1–27.
2. Harriet L. Hartley, "The City Nurse as an Agent for the Prevention of Infant Mortality," in *Transactions of the Nineth Annual Meeting of the American Child Hygiene Association* (Baltimore: Franklin Printing Company, 1919), 122–126.
3. "Women Mob Doctor to Attend Children," undated article from scrapbook of newspaper clippings concerning the influenza epidemic in Philadelphia, College of Physicians of Philadelphia.
4. Harriet L. Hartley, "The Baby in the Epidemic," *Monthly Bulletin of the Department of Public Health and Charities of the City of Philadelphia* 4 (March 1919): 44–45; "Epidemic Statistics," *Monthly Bulletin of the Department of Public Health and Charities of the City of Philadelphia* 4 (March 1919): 46–47.
5. Harriet L. Hartley, "The Baby in the Clinic," *Emergency Service of the Pennsylvania Council of*

National Defense in the Influenza Crisis: Report of The Vice-Director, Department of Medicine, Sanitation and Hospitals (Harrisburg, PA: Pennsylvania Council of National Defense, 1918); "What the Health Department Has Done to Curb the Epidemic of Influenza," *Monthly Bulletin of the Department of Public Health and Charities of the City of Philadelphia* 3 (October–November 1918): 1–27.

6. A. A. Cairns, "Public Health Control of the Influenza Pandemic in Philadelphia," *Monthly Bulletin of the Department of Public Health and Charities of the City of Philadelphia* 4 (March 1919): 34.
7. "Work of the Sisters During the Epidemic of Influenza, October 1918," *Records of the American Catholic Historical Society of Philadelphia*, 30 (March 1919): 28.
8. Hartley, "The Baby in the Epidemic," 45.
9. Patricia M. Lantis and H. Hughes Evans, "Caring for Pandemic Orphans: The Spanish Flu Experience," *Pediatrics* 51 (February 2023): e2021054525.
10. Women's Auxiliary of the Hospital of University of Pennsylvania's Ward G (Children's Ward) Minutes, MC166, Barbara Bates Center for the Study of the History of Nursing, University of Pennsylvania School of Nursing, Philadelphia. Children's names are anonymized. The quotation is from the January 1919 report.
11. "Work of the Sisters," 34.
12. "Philadelphia: How the Social Agencies Organized to Serve the Sick and the Dead," *The Survey* (October 19, 1918): 74–76.
13. *Emergency Service; Southeastern Chapter of the American Red Cross in the Influenza Epidemic September–October 1918* (Philadelphia, PA: American Red Cross, n.d.).
14. *Annual Report for 41st Year October 1, 1918–September 30, 1919, Philadelphia Society for Organizing Charity*, University of Michigan Online Influenza Archive, https://quod.lib.umich.edu/f/flu/6010flu.0016.106 (accessed April 20, 2023).
15. *37th Annual Report of the Children's Aid Society of Pennsylvania for the Year 1918*, University of Michigan Online Influenza Archive, https://quod.lib.umich.edu/f/flu/0670flu.0015.760 (accessed April 20, 2023).
16. Visiting Nurse Society of Philadelphia for the Year Ending December 31, 1918, Barbara Bates Center for the Study of the History of Nursing, University of Pennsylvania School of Nursing, Philadelphia.
17. "Visiting Nurses Busy," *Philadelphia Inquirer*, October 20, 1918, 11.
18. Jeffrey P. Brosco, "Policy and Poverty: Child and Community Health in Philadelphia, 1900–1930," *Archives of Pediatric and Adolescent Medicine* 149 (December 1995): 1381–1387; Cynthia A. Connolly and Janet Golden, "Save 100,000 Babies: The 1918 Children's Year and Its Legacy," *American Journal of Public Health* 108, no. 7 (2018): 902–907.
19. Janet Golden, *Babies Made Us Modern: How Infants Brought Americans into the Twentieth Century* (New York, NY: Cambridge University Press, 2018), 174.
20. Sara J. Rosenbaum, D. Richard Mauery, Peter Shin, and Julia Hidalgo, *National Security and U.S. Child Health Policy: The Origins and Continuing Role of Medicaid and EPSDT* (Washington, DC: Department of Health Policy, School of Public Health and Health Services, George Washington University, 2005).
21. Children First, *COVID's Impact on Children in Philadelphia*, August 2022, https://www.childrenfirstpa.org/news/covids-impact-on-children-in-philadelphia (accessed April 20, 2023).
22. L. Charles Bailey, Hanieh Razzaghi, Evanette K. Burrows, et al., "Assessment of 135 794 Pediatric Patients Tested for Severe Acute Respiratory Syndrome Coronavirus 2 Across the United States," *JAMA Pediatrics* 175, no. 2 (2021): 176–184.
23. Children First, *COVID's Impact*.
24. Ariana Eunjung Cha, "This Is a Crisis: Tens of Thousands of Children Affected by Pandemic-Related Deaths of Parents," *Washington Post*, October 7, 2021.
25. Wendy Ruderman, "Philadelphia's Most Vulnerable Children Suffer Fallout from COVID-19 Crisis," *Philadelphia Inquirer*, April 6, 2020.
26. Siddharth Chandra, Julia Christensen, Svenn-Erik Mamelund, and Nigel Paneth, "Short-Term Birth Sequelae of the 1918–1920 Influenza Pandemic in the United States: State-Level Analysis," *American Journal of Epidemiology* 187, no. 12 (2018): 2585–2595; Douglas Almond and Bhashkar Mazumder, "The 1918 Influenza Pandemic and Subsequent Health Outcomes: An Analysis of SIPP Data," *American Economic Review* 95, no. 2 (2005): 258–262.
27. John McCarthy, Diane Liu, and Frederick Kaskel, "The Need for Life-Course Study of Children Born to Mothers with Prior COVID-19 Infection," *JAMA Pediatrics* 175, no. 11 (2021): 1097–1098.
28. American Rescue Plan Act of 2021, Public Law 117-2, 117th Congress, March 11, 2021, https://www.congress.gov/bill/117th-congress/house-bill/1319/text (accessed April 20, 2023).

State-Level History of Overdose Deaths Involving Stimulants in the United States, 1999–2020

David Kline, PhD, Amanda M. Bunting, PhD, Staci A. Hepler, PhD, Ariadne Rivera-Aguirre, MPP, Noa Krawczyk, PhD, and Magdalena Cerda, DrPH

See also Cooper et al., p. 933.

Objectives. To examine the state-level history of US overdose deaths involving stimulants with and without opioids from 1999 to 2020.

Methods. We used death certificate data from the National Center for Health Statistics to categorize deaths into 4 groups of interest: cocaine with and without opioids, and psychostimulants with and without opioids. We used a Bayesian multiple change point model to describe the timing and magnitude of changes in overdose death rates involving stimulants for each state and year.

Results. There was little change in the death rates of cocaine without opioids. Death rates involving cocaine and opioids sharply increased around 2015, particularly in the Northeast and Mid-Atlantic. We also observed steady increases in deaths involving psychostimulants without opioids just before 2010, particularly in states in the West and South. Deaths involving psychostimulants with opioids increased around 2015 with largest increases concentrated in Appalachian states.

Conclusions. There is significant geographic heterogeneity in the co-involvement of stimulants in the US overdose crisis. Results can inform public health efforts to inform state-level overdose efforts such as naloxone distribution. (*Am J Public Health*. 2023;113(9):991–999. https://doi.org/10.2105/AJPH.2023.307337)

AJPH September 2023, Vol 113, No. 9

The increase of co-involved stimulant and opioid overdoses is a critical public health concern. National data of age-adjusted overdose deaths indicate a nearly 9.4-times increase in psychostimulant and 5.5-times increase in cocaine overdoses that co-involved opioids from 2009 to 2019.[1] As compared with other geographic regions in the United States, the Northeast is reported to experience a particular burden. Data from 2019 indicate a higher percentage of co-involved overdoses occurred in that region (79.6% psychostimulants, 83.1% cocaine).[1]

The nationwide emergence of increasing stimulant use is often referred to as the "fourth wave" of the opioid overdose epidemic. Beyond fatality data, evidence of the fourth wave spans from observed increases in emergency department visits with co-involved opioids and stimulants,[2] drug seizure data,[3] and community-level research studies observing changing drug-use patterns over time.[4] The current fourth wave is particularly fatal because of the co-involvement of opioids and stimulants within the context of the co-occurring rise of synthetic opioids.[5] The driving forces of the new wave are poorly understood, but the current rise of stimulants is entwined with the opioid epidemic in what is increasingly understood as a polydrug and co-use crisis.[6] The fourth wave is uniquely complex given that there are limited interventions for stimulant use.

Provisional overdose data from 2021 report an increase across the United States among overdose fatalities involving synthetic opioids, psychostimulants, and cocaine.[7] However, a homogenous approach across the United States may not be appropriate, as each region and state is grappling with specific stimulant–opioid combinations that may call for different responses. For example, rural areas and the western United States appear to have more notable methamphetamine use as compared with cocaine use in urban areas and the eastern United States.[5,8–10] In previous waves of the opioid crisis, all states were eventually affected, as exampled by synthetic opioid overdoses,[11] which were first greater in the eastern United States, with western states experiencing increases as the wave continued. Some of the regional trends in the current fourth wave have been observed piecemeal (year by year),[12,13] but research has not yet explored state-level variability in the timing and magnitude of changes in the rate of fatal overdoses involving combined opioids and stimulants.

The goal of our study was to examine the state-level history of overdose deaths across the country involving stimulants with and without opioids over a 21-year period. This study builds on previous research that examined geographic variability in opioid crisis outcomes at the subnational (e.g., local, state) level.[14] A systematic review of geographic-based studies of overdose found 20% examined state-level trends at a nationwide level; however, the majority of these used descriptive mapping techniques, and none examined overlapping opioid and stimulant overdose rates.[14] The current research fills a gap both substantively and methodologically through use of descriptive modeling to illuminate state-level overdose mortality trends nationwide involving multiple types of substances. Specifically, we used a Bayesian multiple change point model to flexibly estimate time series for each state and determine when and how rates of overdose death change within each state over time.

METHODS

We used the restricted-use mortality data set[15] from the National Center for Health Statistics to obtain overdose death counts from 1999 to 2020 in the continental United States. Using *International Classification of Disease, Tenth Revision, Second Edition* (*ICD-10*; Geneva, Switzerland: World Health Organization; 2004) codes, we first identified poisoning deaths (X40–44, X60–64, X85, Y10–14) that involved cocaine (T40.5) or psychostimulants (T43.6). Given increasing trends of polysubstance use, we were also interested in deaths that also involved opioids, denoted by the presence of codes T40.0, T40.1, T40.2, T40.3, T40.4, and T40.6.

We then categorized deaths into 4 groups of interest: cocaine without opioids, cocaine with opioids, psychostimulants without opioids, and psychostimulants with opioids. We also conducted a sensitivity analysis that limited the combination with opioids to involvement of synthetic opioids (T40.4). A death involving both cocaine and a psychostimulant would be counted within each group for which it met the definition. Separate groups were not created for the cocaine and psychostimulant combination (9047 deaths across all states and years) because of small counts when broken down by state and year. For each group, deaths were aggregated to the state level by year of death. We used annual state population estimates from CDC WONDER[16] to calculate mortality rates. To account for potential regional structure, we obtained the Centers for Medicare and Medicaid Services region (Appendix Table A, available as a supplement to the online version of this article at https://ajph.org) for each state to use as a covariate.

Our primary goal for this analysis was to describe the timing and magnitude of changes within states for crude overdose death rates involving stimulants over time. This is important as rates have both increased and decreased during the time period studied across different states, and all states do not follow a similar common functional form. We used a Bayesian multiple change point model that allowed us to flexibly estimate state-specific time series without prespecifying a functional form or the number of change points, account for hierarchical structure and multivariate dependence across groups, and fully quantify uncertainty within a single unified model.

For each state, year, and drug group, we assumed the death counts were Poisson distributed with mean determined by the product of the state's total population in that year and a rate parameter (i.e., the death rate for that drug group). For each state and drug group, we assumed the rate parameter to be constant over time until an estimated change point occurred. When an estimated change point occurred, we estimated a new rate parameter for that state and drug group, and it remained constant for subsequent years until another change point occurred. To align with existing statistical literature,[17] we defined each change in the rate parameter as a "regime change." That is, we defined a regime as the set of years for a state and drug type that share a common death rate parameter. The regime changed when we estimated that a change point occurred and the rate parameter had changed.

Statistically, our model provided very flexible, semiparametric estimates of the complex trends associated with mortality in each drug group in each state. Practically, our model enabled us to estimate time series for state- and drug-specific mortality rates and to explicitly estimate the timing and magnitude of change. Conceptually, we believed the underlying structure of changes in rates determined by multiple change points better fits the true epidemiological process that governs fluctuation in rates of overdose deaths by drug type, which may be related to abrupt changes in illicit drug supply, policy, enforcement, and other social environmental conditions. While this structure included the possibility for exponential growth, it provided a more general and flexible approach than strictly assuming exponential growth as is common for infectious diseases.

To model whether a change point occurred, we assumed a binary indicator of whether a given year was a change point for each state and drug type. We assumed the probability of a change point followed a centered autologistic model[18] with a regional random effect. We used the autologistic model to capture temporal dependence in the probability of a change within a state and drug group. The regional random effect implied that the log odds of change point for states in the same Centers for Medicare and Medicaid Services region may be correlated, and we assumed a multivariate structure for the random effect to capture dependence across drug groups within a region.

In practice, we interpreted the probability that there was a change to be a measure of volatility in the death rate. That is, higher probabilities of change signified that there were more likely to be change points and changing death rates (i.e., a volatile rather than a stable process in time). Within this context, the autologistic model implied that states with more volatility were more likely to remain volatile, and states with more stability were more likely to remain stable. Likewise, the regional random effect implied that collective regional volatility would impact the volatility of each state within the region and that change in one drug group may be related to change in other drug groups, which may reflect changes in the underlying drug supply and market. We believed these assumptions were reasonable and enabled a borrowing of strength within region and over time.

We fit the model within the Bayesian paradigm and assigned prior distributions. For all model parameters, we assumed diffuse, proper prior distributions. We ran a Markov chain Monte Carlo algorithm for 500 000 iterations using the NIMBLE package in R (R Foundation for Statistical Computing, Vienna, Austria).[19] The first 250 000 iterations were discarded as burn-in, and we thinned the remaining samples by 50. We assessed convergence visually using trace plots. The full statistical specification of the model and R code are included in the Appendix (available as a supplement to the online version of this article at https://ajph.org).

RESULTS

In this section and in Appendix Figures A–E, estimates are shown from the model that describe the time series, timing, and magnitude of changes in the death rates involving cocaine with and without opioids and psychostimulants with and without opioids. Figure 1 shows the posterior median estimates of the time series of death rates per 100 000 residents for each state in panels arranged geographically. Rates for West Virginia and Washington, DC, in 2020 exceeded the vertical axis of Figure 1 and are shown in Appendix Figure A. Figure 2 shows posterior median estimates of the death rates in which each row is the time series for a given state, and the rows are sorted from states in the Northeast to the West Coast to highlight large-scale geographic patterns. Appendix Figure B replicates Figure 2 with scales specific to each drug group to better highlight within-group variation.

We observed some general themes across the country during this time period. There was generally little change in the death rates of cocaine without opioids over time across the country with slightly higher rates in the mid- to late 2000s and the late 2010s. Death rates involving cocaine without opioids in Washington, DC, were notably higher than in the rest of the country. Death rates involving cocaine and opioids sharply increased around 2015, particularly in states in the Northeast and Mid-Atlantic. We also saw steady increases in deaths involving psychostimulants without opioids starting just before 2010 and continuing through 2020, particularly in states in the West and South. As with deaths involving cocaine and opioids, we saw sharp increases in deaths involving psychostimulants with opioids starting just before 2015 with some of the largest increases concentrated in Appalachian states like West Virginia, Kentucky, Tennessee, and Ohio. Death rates involving cocaine with opioids were generally higher in the earlier years studied than rates of psychostimulants with opioids, but rates in both groups rapidly increased around the time that fentanyl became more prevalent in the illicit drug supply. A sensitivity analysis limiting deaths involving opioids to only synthetic opioids confirms that they were the primary driver of these increases (analyses not shown).

There also was significant geographic heterogeneity in the evolution of overdose involving stimulants. Figures 1 and 2 illustrate that the northeast

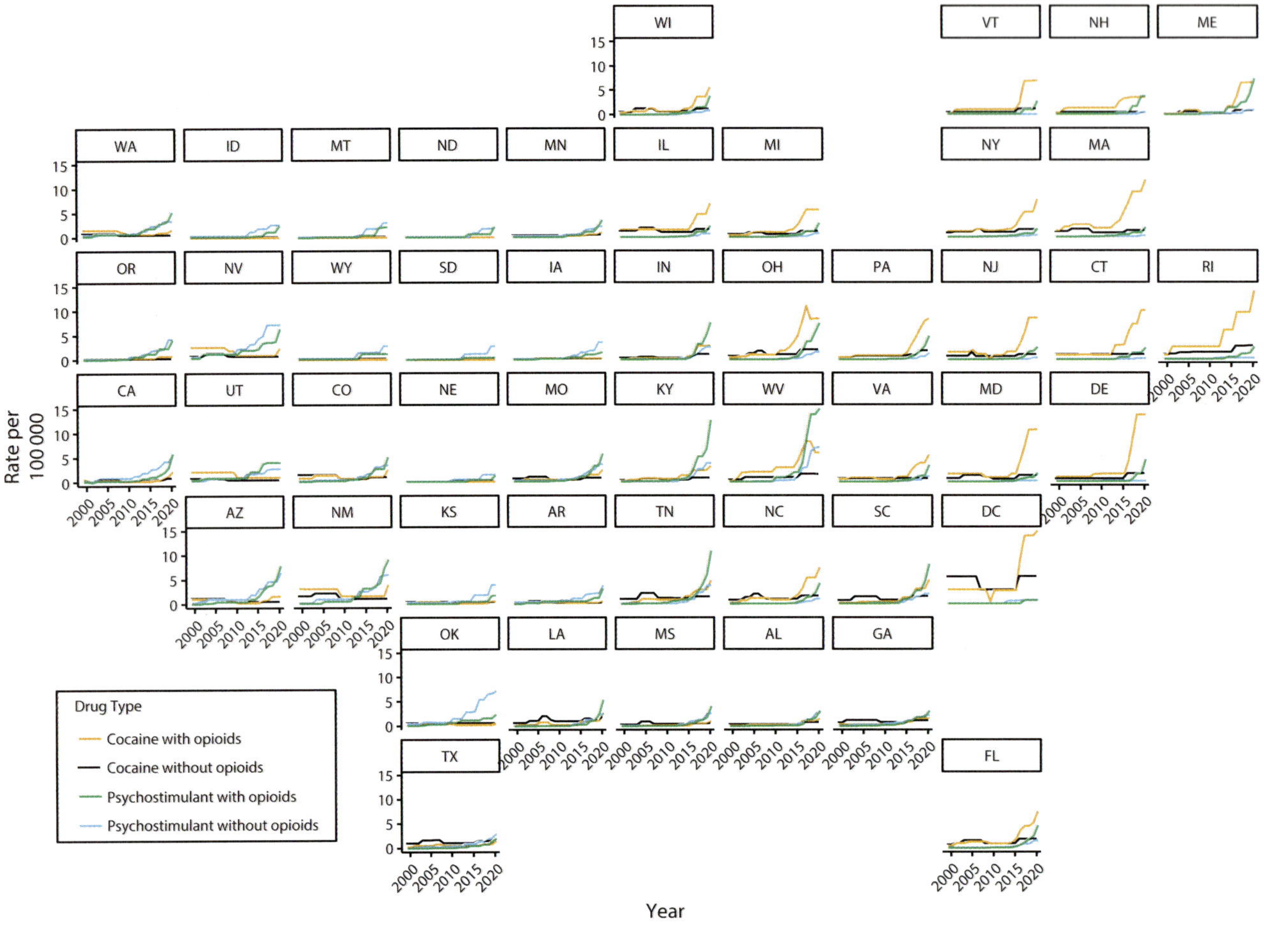

FIGURE 1— Estimates of the Overdose Death Rates per 100 000 Residents: United States, 1999–2020

Note. Vertical axis is truncated at 15 per 100 000. Full series for West Virginia and Washington, DC, are available in Appendix Figure A.

quadrant of the country experienced the highest death rates involving cocaine with opioids, although rates were also increasing into the Midwest. We generally did not observe similar increases in the southern or western parts of the country, with the exception of Florida. In contrast, rates involving psychostimulants with and without opioids primarily increased across the western part of the country and, after 2015, in Appalachian states such as West Virginia, Tennessee, and Kentucky. While rates of death involving psychostimulants both with and without opioids have been increasing, death rates involving psychostimulants with opioids increased the most in West Virginia, Kentucky, Tennessee, Ohio, Indiana, and South Carolina. In the western states, death rates involving psychostimulants with and without opioids followed similar trends. New Mexico, Arizona, and Nevada had some of the highest estimated death rates involving psychostimulants with and without opioids of the western states. Death rates involving psychostimulants without opioids in Oklahoma were relatively high while death rates involving psychostimulants with opioids remained relatively low. Notably, we observed high rates and increasing trends for both cocaine with opioids and psychostimulants with opioids in Ohio, West Virginia, and, to a lesser extent, Pennsylvania, whereas most other states were more concentrated with either cocaine with opioids or psychostimulants with opioids.

Appendix Figure C shows the relative risk of death compared with the previous year for each state and drug type. This figure highlights the timing, direction, and magnitude of change in the death rates. There is little variation in the annual change of the rates involving cocaine without opioids. There is more variation in the timing of increases in rates involving cocaine with opioids after 2015, primarily in the

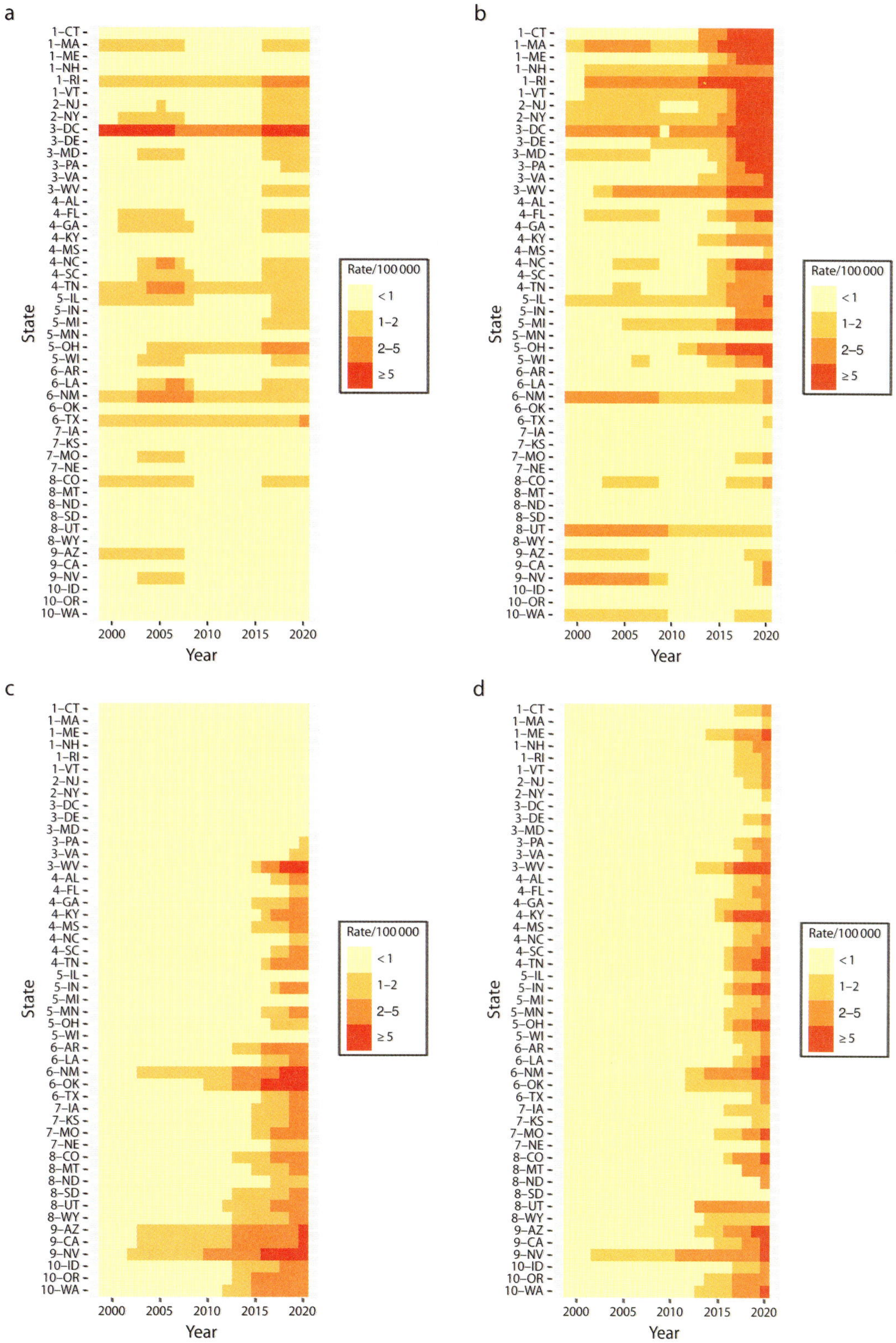

FIGURE 2— Estimated Overdose Death Rates per 100 000 Residents From (a) Cocaine Without Opioids, (b) Cocaine With Opioids, (c) Psychostimulants Without Opioids, and (d) Psychostimulants With Opioids: United States, 1999–2020

Note. Sites are sorted by Centers for Medicare and Medicaid Services region.

eastern half of the country. There is much more widespread variation in the annual changes in rates involving psychostimulants with and without opioids with widespread increases in both primarily after 2013.

Estimates of the log odds of the occurrence of a change point shown in Figure 3 further illuminate trends in the timing of changes. Each point represents the posterior median estimate of the log odds for a state, and the color indicates a greater than 90% posterior probability that the rate increased (red) or decreased (blue) at the change point. For cocaine without opioids, Figure 3a shows relative stability with some states experiencing increased

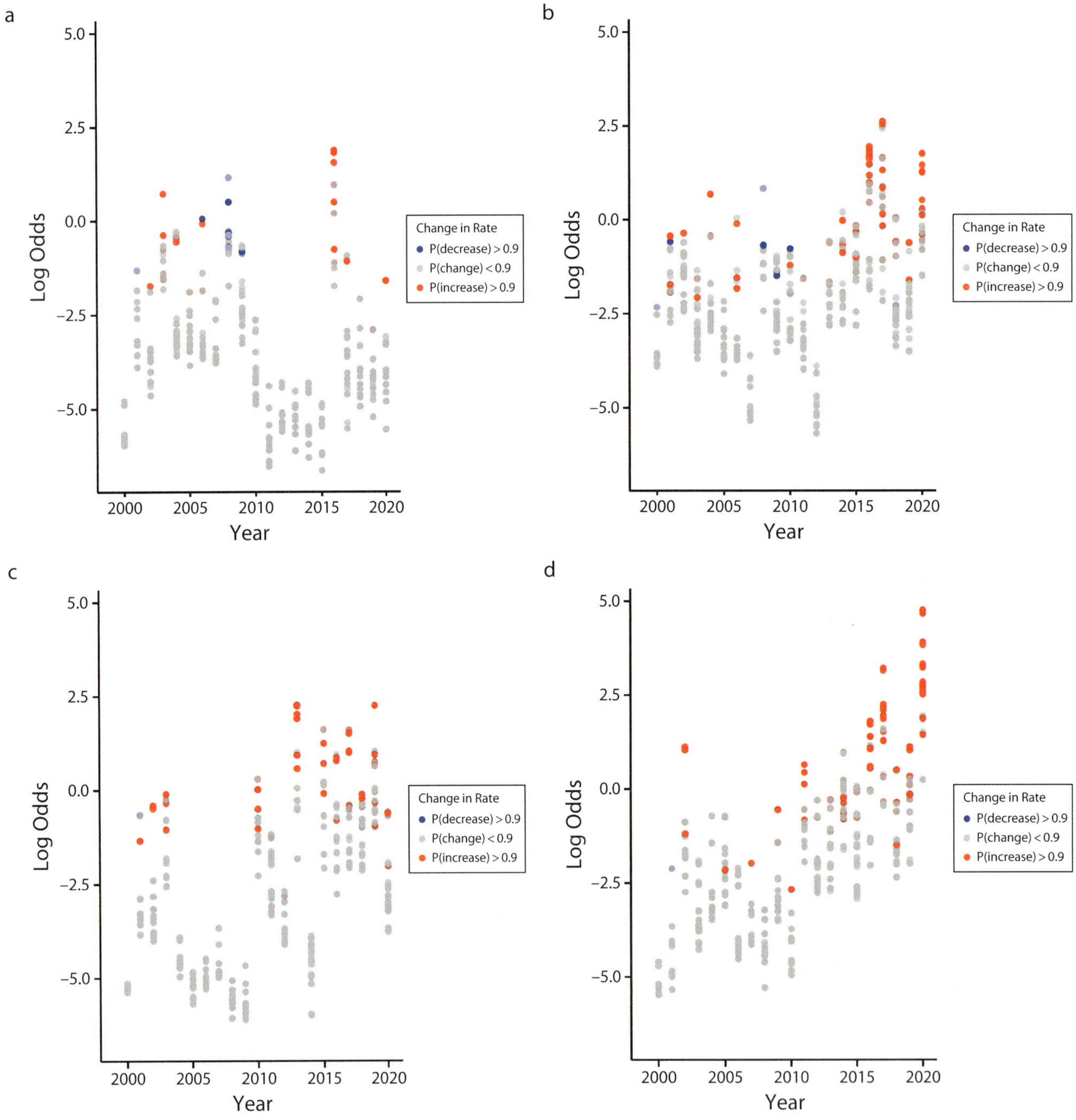

FIGURE 3— Estimated Log Odds of a Change in the Overdose Death Rate for Each US State From 1999–2020

Note. Red points represent a posterior probability that the death rate increased from the previous year of greater than 0.9 and blue points represent a posterior probability that the rate decreased from the previous year of greater than 0.9.

rates in 2016. Figure 3b shows much more volatility (higher log odds of change) after 2015 with the vast majority of changes leading to increased death rates. Figure 3c shows volatility in some states from around 2010 to 2020 with changes tending to be increases in the death rate. Similarly, Figure 3d shows a lot of volatility, particularly after 2015. Estimates of the regional random effects are shown in Appendix Figure D. These findings align with what was observed in Figure 1 but help to more clearly identify trends related to the timing and direction of changes in the death rates for each drug type.

To better visualize geographic heterogeneity across drug groups and time, 2 time series animations are included in Figure E (available as a supplement to the online version of this article at https://ajph.org), highlighting posterior median estimates of the death rates per 100 000 residents and log relative risk of death compared with the previous year. States are outlined if the posterior probability was greater than 0.9 that the rate increased (red) or decreased (blue). Both animations further reinforce the themes observed in the static figures and highlight the degree of geographic heterogeneity that exists across time and drug group.

DISCUSSION

We examined a national state-level history of overdose deaths involving stimulants and found increases in stimulant-involved overdoses, with specific geographic differences. Deaths involving cocaine with opioids increased starting in 2010, with increases observed in the Northeast and Mid-Atlantic states. At the same time, we observed increases in psychostimulant overdoses in the western and southern states. In 2015, psychostimulant overdoses with opioids increased further, most notably in Appalachian regions.

The national examination of state-level overdose trends and Bayesian methodology provided a more nuanced consideration of stimulant–opioid overdose fatalities. Compared with previous cross-sectional and regionally clustered work[1,2] our study demonstrated that examining states outside of their census regions and across time provides insights to subregional differences of substance-specific patterns that may previously have been overlooked. For example, 2016–2017 research clustered at the census regions indicated increases in psychostimulant overdoses involving opioids in Midwestern states,[2] yet 2019 data reported the greatest percentage of these deaths in the Northeast.[1] The current data revealed that the Northeast continues to be heavily impacted by cocaine-involved overdoses. When we examined trends with the statistical techniques used in this study, as opposed to age-adjusted percentages alone, we saw that the Northeast remained more heavily affected by cocaine and opioid–involved overdoses. Furthermore, the tendency for previous research to cluster by region omitted important heterogeneity within regions, such as the current finding that deaths involving cocaine without opioids are substantially higher in Washington, DC, than the rest of the country, and insights into specific Midwestern states where most of the region's deaths are occurring.

The current study's in-depth view of each state's opioid–stimulant overdose profile provides a clear view of the division between states related to the type of stimulant driving overdose fatalities. The increase of psychostimulant overdoses began in 2010 in western and southern states, with increases in co-involved opioid and psychostimulant overdoses starting in 2015 in Appalachian regions. The timing of these overdose fatalities trends similarly to changes in the manufacturing of methamphetamine. Methamphetamine in the United States was previously dominated by a pseudoephedrine method, but changes to laws in the United States in 2006 and Mexico in 2007 were intended to impact supply by regulating the ingredient pseudoephedrine.[20,21] Methamphetamine manufacturing began transitioning to what is known as the P2P (phenyl-2-propanone) method such that, by 2010, seized samples that used the P2P method were greater than the number of samples with the pseudoephedrine method, and, by 2015, the pseudoephedrine method appeared to be extinct.[20] Related to these manufacturing changes, the purity of methamphetamine increased.[20]

While methamphetamine is available in all states, the Drug Enforcement Administration reports the highest availability in the West and Midwest.[22] The changes to the methamphetamine process and subsequent increased purity may relate to the observed trends observed in overdoses, and further research should explore the effects of these policies on overdoses. Notably, disproportionate harms from the opioid epidemic first began in Appalachian areas,[23] and the current analyses ring the alarm that attention must be paid to the struggles of Appalachia if methamphetamine's contribution to the current overdose crisis can be abated.

Cocaine-involved overdoses appear to be geographically distinct from psychostimulant deaths. The increased rate of cocaine-involved overdoses with opioids in the Northeast and Mid-Atlantic since 2015, and the fact that these deaths (along with psychostimulants) are driven by synthetic opioids, is troubling as it leaves intentionality of opioid use unknown. Deaths involving cocaine and opioids may be higher in these regions as they have higher prevalence of fentanyl in drug markets.[24] If the co-use of opioids with stimulants is unintentional, as in the case of fentanyl contamination, individuals may not be aware of the potential benefits of naloxone, the medication that can reverse opioid overdoses. No similar drug exists for stimulant overdoses, and the current overdose crisis has called for an "agnostic" approach to overdose-related respiratory depression.[25] Research of syringe service providers across the nation found lower distribution of naloxone in the eastern United States.[26] While public health entities and researchers have been calling for expanded access of naloxone to persons who use stimulants, it is unclear how naloxone distribution efforts are targeted to this population. Furthermore, individuals at risk for overdose may only have occasional or recreational drug use and be less likely to come into contact with public health messaging or agencies who traditionally target individuals with substance use disorders.

The current research highlights the geographic heterogeneity of the current overdose trends. This information can be used to inform state-level efforts, such as understanding the substances that should be targeted in different public health campaigns. In addition, state leadership may benefit from a state-level view to understand which states are similar to their own so that government groups, nonprofits, and coalitions of persons who use drugs from similarly situated states can work together. Furthermore, an understanding of which stimulant drives overdose in each state can assist in efforts to expand naloxone access. Additional research may also consider exploring the treatment and policy landscape in states that are disparate in their patterns (e.g., the District of Columbia, Oklahoma, and West Virginia). While more research is needed to understand if opioid use with psychostimulants and cocaine is intentional, communities should consider how to reach populations using stimulants that may not obtain naloxone through more typical routes of access (e.g., syringe service programs, opioid medication programs). AJPH

ABOUT THE AUTHORS

David Kline is with the Department of Biostatistics and Data Science, Wake Forest University (WFU) School of Medicine, Winston-Salem, NC. Amanda M. Bunting, Ariadne Rivera-Aguirre, Noa Krawczyk, and Magdalena Cerda are with the Center for Opioid Epidemiology and Policy, Department of Population Health, New York University (NYU) Langone School of Medicine, New York, NY. Staci A. Hepler is with the Department of Statistical Sciences, Wake Forest University.

CORRESPONDENCE

Correspondence should be sent to Amanda M. Bunting, 180 Madison Ave, New York, NY 10016 (e-mail: amanda.bunting@nyulangone.org). Reprints can be ordered at https://ajph.org by clicking the "Reprints" link.

PUBLICATION INFORMATION

Full Citation: Kline D, Bunting AM, Hepler SA, Rivera-Aguirre A, Krawczyk N, Cerda M. State-level history of overdose deaths involving stimulants in the United States, 1999–2020. *Am J Public Health*. 2023;113(9):991–999.

Acceptance Date: May 11, 2023.

DOI: https://doi.org/10.2105/AJPH.2023.307337

CONTRIBUTORS

D. Kline and A. M. Bunting contributed equally. D. Kline contributed to conceptualization, methodology, formal analysis, visualization, and writing the original draft. A. M. Bunting contributed to conceptualization, methodology, and writing the original draft. S. A. Hepler contributed to conceptualization, methodology, formal analysis, and review and editing of the article. A. Rivera-Aguirre contributed to data curation and review and editing of the article. N. Krawczyk contributed to conceptualization and review and editing of the article. M. Cerda contributed to conceptualization, methodology, resources, and review and editing of the article.

ACKNOWLEDGMENTS

Research reported in this publication was supported by the National Institute on Drug Abuse of the National Institutes of Health under awards R01DA052214, R25DA037190, and K01DA053435.

A preliminary version of this research was presented at the NYU Polysubstance Use Symposium on October 20, 2022.

Computations were performed using the WFU High Performance Computing Facility, a centrally managed computational resource available to WFU researchers including faculty, staff, students, and collaborators.

Note: The content is solely the responsibility of the authors and does not necessarily represent the official views of the National Institutes of Health.

CONFLICTS OF INTEREST

N. Krawczyk and M. Cerda are involved in ongoing opioid litigation. Other authors have no conflicts of interest to declare.

HUMAN PARTICIPANT PROTECTION

This research is not human participant research.

REFERENCES

1. Hedegaard H. Co-involvement of opioids in drug overdose deaths involving cocaine and psychostimulants. NCHS data brief; no. 406. Hyattsville, MD: National Center for Health Statistics; 2021. https://doi.org/10.15620/cdc:103966
2. Hoots B, Vivolo-Kantor A, Seth P. The rise in non-fatal and fatal overdoses involving stimulants with and without opioids in the United States. *Addiction.* 2020;115(5):946–958. https://doi.org/10.1111/add.14878
3. Jones CM, Bekheet F, Park JN, Alexander GC. The evolving overdose epidemic: synthetic opioids and rising stimulant-related harms. *Epidemiol Rev.* 2020;42(1):154–166. https://doi.org/10.1093/epirev/mxaa011
4. Palamar JJ, Han BH, Keyes KM. Trends in characteristics of individuals who use methamphetamine in the United States, 2015–2018. *Drug Alcohol Depend.* 2020;213:108089. https://doi.org/10.1016/j.drugalcdep.2020.108089
5. Mattson CL. Trends and geographic patterns in drug and synthetic opioid overdose deaths—United States, 2013–2019. *MMWR Morb Mortal Wkly Rep.* 2021;70(6):202–207. https://doi.org/10.15585/mmwr.mm7006a4
6. Ciccarone D. The rise of illicit fentanyls, stimulants and the fourth wave of the opioid overdose crisis. *Curr Opin Psychiatry.* 2021;34(4):344–350. https://doi.org/10.1097/YCO.0000000000000717
7. Centers for Disease Control and Prevention, National Center for Health Statistics. US overdose

deaths in 2021 increased half as much as in 2020—but are still up 15%. May 11, 2022. Available at: https://www.cdc.gov/nchs/pressroom/nchs_press_releases/2022/202205.htm. Accessed December 12, 2022.

8. Jones CM, Compton WM, Mustaquim D. Patterns and characteristics of methamphetamine use among adults—United States, 2015–2018. *MMWR Morb Mortal Wkly Rep.* 2020;69(12):317–323. https://doi.org/10.15585/mmwr.mm6912a1

9. Kerridge BT, Chou SP, Pickering RP, et al. Changes in the prevalence and correlates of cocaine use and cocaine use disorder in the United States, 2001–2002 and 2012–2013. *Addict Behav.* 2019;90:250–257. https://doi.org/10.1016/j.addbeh.2018.11.005

10. Hedegaard H, Bastian BA, Trinidad JP, et al. Regional differences in the drugs most frequently involved in drug overdose deaths: United States, 2017. *Natl Vital Stat Rep.* 2019;68(12):1–16. Available at: https://stacks.cdc.gov/view/cdc/82186. Accessed April 17, 2023.

11. Scholl L, Seth P, Kariisa M, Wilson N, Baldwin G. Drug and opioid-involved overdose deaths—United States, 2013–2017. *MMWR Morb Mortal Wkly Rep.* 2018;67(5152):1419–1427. https://doi.org/10.15585/mmwr.mm6751521e1

12. Gladden RM. Changes in opioid-involved overdose deaths by opioid type and presence of benzodiazepines, cocaine, and methamphetamine—25 states, July–December 2017 to January–June 2018. *MMWR Morb Mortal Wkly Rep.* 2019; 68(34):737–744. https://doi.org/10.15585/mmwr.mm6834a2

13. O'Donnell J. Vital Signs: Characteristics of drug overdose deaths involving opioids and stimulants—24 states and the District of Columbia, January–June 2019. *MMWR Morb Mortal Wkly Rep.* 2020;69(35):1189–1197. https://doi.org/10.15585/mmwr.mm6935a1

14. Sauer J, Stewart K. Geographic information science and the United States opioid overdose crisis: a scoping review of methods, scales, and application areas. *Soc Sci Med.* 2023;317:115525. https://doi.org/10.1016/j.socscimed.2022.115525

15. National Center for Health Statistics. Restricted-use vital statistics data. March 25, 2022. Available at: https://www.cdc.gov/nchs/nvss/nvss-restricted-data.htm. Accessed April 6, 2022.

16. Centers for Disease Control and Prevention, National Center for Health Statistics. Bridged-race population estimates 1990–2020 request. Bridged-race population estimates, United States July 1st resident population by state, county, age, sex, bridged-race, and Hispanic origin. CDC WONDER online database. Available at: https://wonder.cdc.gov/Bridged-Race-v2020.HTML. Accessed August 29, 2022.

17. Ko SIM, Chong TTL, Ghosh P. Dirichlet process hidden Markov multiple change-point model. *Bayesian Analysis.* 2015;10(2):275–296. https://doi.org/10.1214/14-BA910

18. Caragea PC, Kaiser M. Autologistic models with interpretable parameters. *J Agric Biol Environ Stat.* 2009;14(3):281–300. https://doi.org/10.1198/jabes.2009.07032

19. de Valpine P, Turek D, Paciorek CJ, Anderson-Bergman C, Lang DT, Bodik R. Programming with models: writing statistical algorithms for general model structures with NIMBLE. *J Comput Graph Stat.* 2017;26(2):403–413. https://doi.org/10.1080/10618600.2016.1172487

20. Toske SG, McKibben TD. Monitoring methamphetamine in the United States: a two-decade review as seen by the DEA methamphetamine profiling program. *Drug Test Anal.* 2022;14(3):416–426. https://doi.org/10.1002/dta.3186

21. Drug Enforcement Administration. Retail sales of scheduled listed chemical products; self-certification of regulated sellers of scheduled listed chemical products. Interim final rule with request for comment. *Fed Regist.* 2006;71(186):56008–56027.

22. Drug Enforcement Administration. 2020 national drug threat assessment. 2021. DEA-DCT-DIR-008-21. Available at: https://www.dea.gov/sites/default/files/2021-02/DIR-008-21%202020%20National%20Drug%20Threat%20Assessment_WEB.pdf. Accessed November 9, 2022.

23. National Association of Counties and Appalachian Regional Commission. Opioids in Appalachia. 2019. Available at: https://www.naco.org/sites/default/files/documents/Opioids-Full.pdf. Accessed November 9, 2022.

24. Zoorob M. Fentanyl shock: the changing geography of overdose in the United States. *Int J Drug Policy.* 2019;70:40–46. https://doi.org/10.1016/j.drugpo.2019.04.010

25. Pergolizzi JV, Dahan A, LeQuang JA, Raffa RB. The conundrum of polysubstance overdose. *J Clin Pharm Ther.* 2021;46(5):1189–1193. https://doi.org/10.1111/jcpt.13362

26. Lambdin BH, Bluthenthal RN, Wenger LD, et al. Overdose education and naloxone distribution within syringe service programs—United States, 2019. *MMWR Morb Mortal Wkly Rep.* 2020;69(33):1117–1121. https://doi.org/10.15585/mmwr.mm6933a2

Diversity of the US Public Health Workforce Pipeline (2016–2020): Role of Academic Institutions

Anushree Vichare, PhD, MPH, MBBS, Yoon Hong Park, MPP, and Christine M. Plepys, MS

See also Kapadia, p. 936.

Objectives. To develop a diversity index (DI) comparing the diversity of graduates across public health schools and programs in the United States and to examine characteristics associated with institutions' graduate diversity.

Methods. We analyzed longitudinal data from the Association of Schools and Programs of Public Health (ASPPH) across 5 academic years (2016–2017 to 2020–2021) for 109 ASPPH members. The outcome was the percentage of underrepresented minority (URM) students among those with bachelor's and graduate degrees in public health. The DI was constructed by dividing the percentage of URM graduates by the percentage of URM residents 20 to 35 years of age in the state where the ASPPH member was located.

Results. The mean DI score increased from 0.7 in 2016 to 0.8 in 2020, but URM students remain underrepresented. A 1-percentage-point increase in the proportion of URM faculty members was associated with a 0.7-percentage-point increase in the proportion of URM graduates ($P < .001$).

Conclusions. Although the diversity of the public health educational pipeline shows an upward trend, racial/ethnic minority students remain underrepresented in public health. We found that institutional characteristics such as faculty diversity, program degree level, and area of study were associated with student diversity. (*Am J Public Health*. 2023;113(9):1000–1008. https://doi.org/10.2105/AJPH.2023.307352)

AJPH September 2023, Vol 113, No. 9

Despite improvements in health indicators, racial and ethnic disparities continue to remain a public health challenge. COVID-19 brought to the surface existing structural racism that widened gaps in access to care and health outcomes, disproportionately affecting racial and ethnic minorities.[1,2] A racially and ethnically diverse workforce can be instrumental in addressing existing disparities.[3,4] Diversity represents heterogeneity in terms of class, race, ethnicity, and sexual identity and is a key indicator of workforce development.

There is widespread agreement that more representative workforces are better able to serve diverse populations.[5,6] Yet, the federal, state, and local public health workforce is not diverse and is underrepresented racially and ethnically at the supervisory and managerial levels. For example, the 2017 Public Health Workforce Interests and Needs Survey suggests that the workforce in the public sector is not representative of the nation; 59% of the workforce is White, compared with 16% non-Hispanic Black and 13% Hispanic.[7–9]

Lack of diversity in the public health workforce can occur as a result of myriad factors, including underrepresentation of marginalized groups in the public health education pipeline. There has been substantial growth in the degrees conferred in public health, but the growth of Black and Hispanic representation has not kept pace.[10–12] Over the past 20 years, the proportion of racial and ethnic minority representation has increased by less than 5 percentage points for graduate student enrollment and by less than 3 percentage points among tenured faculty.[13]

Increases in racial/ethnic diversity among students, graduates, and faculty in public health schools and programs can contribute to parallel increases in the diversity of the public health workforce. Thus, public health educational institutions play a significant role in prioritizing admission strategies to recruit public health students with diverse backgrounds and offering an environment with strong mentoring, advising, and skill development. However, research in this area has not examined institutional-level diversity and has been limited in providing an understanding of the role public health institutions play in the enrollment and retention of students from disadvantaged groups.

Evaluating student diversity at the institution level is important and socially relevant. Decisions about student admissions are made at the institutional level, and it seems logical that different types of academic institutions have different profiles that can affect the diversity of the student body.[14] Existing research has focused on the benefits of diversity in the context of a university, barriers to increasing diversity, ways to increase and maintain diversity, and, more recently, the importance of ethnic and cultural diversity to regional economic growth and innovation.[15] Here we attempt to contribute to the existing evidence by exploring a metric to track improvements in student diversity at the public health institutional level. We also build on current evidence by assessing the impact of institutional characteristics on student diversity. In our study, diversity is defined in terms of race and ethnicity as a result of issues regarding data availability.

Our study's objectives were two fold. First, we sought to create an institutional-level diversity index (DI) by comparing the diversity of public health graduates with the diversity of US residents between the ages of 20 and 35 years (the general age range of public health graduates).[16] Our second objective was to evaluate the relative contributions of characteristics such as ownership status, geographic location, faculty diversity, and student body diversity at public health educational institutions.

The findings from our study provide a data-driven strategy to track diversity at the institutional level via the DI and explore factors associated with increased diversity in the educational pipeline. This can potentially inform future investments and recruitment and retention strategies to improve the diversity of the public health educational pipeline and eventually the public health workforce. The DI, a diversity statistic, will also potentially enable cross comparisons of diversity between institutions of higher public health education in the United States. In addition, it will provide a diversity "benchmark" that compares the racial and ethnic composition of the student body relative to the racial and ethnic composition of the institution's catchment or service area. Public health workforce shortages are likely to worsen over time, with a potential loss of about 57% of the governmental workforce by 2025.[17] With calls for investments in building a sustainable workforce, the opportunity to increase the representation of underrepresented minority (URM) individuals is well timed.

METHODS

We derived our primary data from the Association of Schools and Programs of Public Health (ASPPH), which had information available on each of its former and current member schools and programs for 5 academic years (2016–2017 to 2020–2021). ASPPH represents 142 schools that are accredited or have applied to be accredited by the Council on Education for Public Health (of approximately 260 schools and programs conferring public health degrees). Our information came from ASPPH's annual data on faculty, annual data on the student life cycle (i.e., applications, acceptances, enrollments, graduations), and directory of members and their institutional characteristics. Specifically, our data comprised information on (1) student cohorts' composition according to race/ethnicity, citizenship, degree level (bachelor's, master's, doctoral), area of study, and degree delivery type (campus based, distance learning, executive format); (2) faculty racial/ethnic composition; and (3) each school or program's zip code, ownership, and institutional type (public health program or school of public health).

We also used American Community Survey data from 2016 to 2020 to estimate the diversity of the population in the state where each school or program was located, 2010 US Department of Agriculture Rural–Urban Commuting Area Codes to determine the rurality of schools and programs, and the National Center for Education Statistics Integrated Postsecondary Education Data System to identify historically Black colleges and universities. We excluded schools and programs if the total number of US citizen graduates was less than 10 or data on faculty and graduate race/ethnicity were missing (Figure A, available as a supplement to the online version of this article at http://www.ajph.org). Our analytic sample included 806 observations from 109 schools and programs located in 41 US states and the District of Columbia.

Black, Hispanic, American Indian/Alaska Native, and Native Hawaiian/Pacific Islander populations are recognized as being historically underrepresented in science, technology, engineering, and mathematics talent pools.[18,19] We therefore defined these racial/ethnic groups as URM groups. To track the diversity of graduates relative to the diversity of the population in the state where each school or program is located, we constructed the DI for each school or program in each year for each degree level by dividing the percentage of URM students among domestic graduates by the percentage of URM students among state residents 20 to 35 years of age. We selected the 20- to 35-year age range because it was the most common range among graduates included in the ASPPH data.

We first plotted a trend line for the average DI of the entire analytic sample and separate trend lines for the 3 degree levels. Next, we tested the associations between students, faculty, and school or program characteristics and student diversity. The key dependent variable for this analysis was the percentage of URM students among domestic graduates overall. Given the relatively intuitive interpretation for a percentage versus an index in a regression model, we used the percentage of URM students as our primary dependent variable rather than the DI.

The explanatory variables included the percentages of the following:

(1) URM individuals among the population 20 to 35 years old in the state where each school or program was located;
(2) international students among graduates;
(3) domestic graduates who earned degrees via distance learning;
(4) domestic graduates with degrees in 1 of the 6 main areas of study (biostatistics, epidemiology, general public health, global health, maternal and child health, and health policy and management);
(5) full-time equivalents among URM faculty members;
(6) faculty members of unspecified race/ethnicity;
(7) types of school and program ownership (private vs public); and
(8) types of institutions (schools vs programs of public health).

We clustered standard errors at the school or program level so that observations across different degree levels in different years would be correlated within the same school or program.

We used pooled ordinary least squares models for our main analysis but conducted robustness checks with school or program random effects and year fixed effects to account for time-invariant unobservable secular trends. We also conducted subgroup analyses by bachelor's and graduate degree levels. Finally, to account for the relationship between the diversity of graduates and the diversity of applicants, we added the diversity of applicants 2 to 3 years before a graduation year to the main model. In our extended analyses, we focused on master's degrees programs given the relatively fixed length of the academic cycle in comparison with bachelor's and doctoral degree programs.

RESULTS

Of the 109 schools and programs in our analytic sample, almost one third (n = 37) were private (Table 1). Whereas all schools and programs conferred master's degrees, less than half conferred bachelor's degrees (41%) or doctoral degrees (40%). The majority of schools and programs were located in metropolitan core areas (94%); none were in rural areas. No school in our sample was officially recognized as a historically Black college or university according to the Integrated Postsecondary Education Data System.

The mean DI score was 0.78 (Table 2), implying continued underrepresentation of URM students relative to school or program's state racial/ethnic composition. Although mean DI scores for Black, Native Hawaiian/Pacific Islander, and American Indian/Alaska Native graduates were above 1, the score for Hispanic graduates was less than 1 (mean = 0.59). We also found that racial/ethnic minority faculty members continue to be underrepresented in public health. The mean percentage of URM faculty members was 14% (9% Black and 5% Hispanic).

Diversity Index Trend Analysis

The mean DI trend line suggested gradual improvements in diversity among graduates over time (Figure 1). For example, the 2014 mean DI score of 0.7 increased to slightly more than 0.8 in 2020. However, the mean score was still less than 1, implying underrepresentation of URM graduates relative to the population they would serve. Furthermore, we found differences by degree level; the mean DI score was higher for bachelor's degrees (0.98) than for master's (0.82) or doctoral (0.62) degrees.

Regression Analysis

Regression results from our ordinary least squares model (model 1) and

TABLE 1— Characteristics of ASPPH Member Schools and Programs in the Analytic Sample: United States, 2016–2020

Characteristic	Schools/Programs (n = 109), No. (%)	Observations (n = 806), No. (%)
Ownership type		
Private	37 (33.94)	215 (26.67)
Public	72 (66.06)	591 (73.33)
Institution type		
Public health program	48 (44.04)	178 (22.08)
School of public health	61 (55.96)	628 (77.92)
Degree level[a]		
Bachelor's	45 (41.28)	185 (22.95)
Master's	109 (100.00)	454 (56.33)
Doctoral	44 (40.37)	167 (20.72)
Institution location		
Metropolitan area core	103 (93.50)	781 (96.90)
Metropolitan area high commuting	2 (1.83)	2 (0.25)
Micropolitan area core	4 (3.67)	23 (2.85)
Rural area	0 (0.00)	0 (0.00)
Historically Black college or university	0 (0.00)	0 (0.00)
Year[b]		
2016	78 (71.56)	144 (17.87)
2017	87 (79.82)	153 (18.98)
2018	95 (87.16)	166 (20.60)
2019	97 (88.99)	170 (21.09)
2020	97 (88.99)	173 (21.46)

Note. ASPPH = Association of Schools and Programs of Public Health.

[a]The number of schools for each degree level does not sum to the total number of schools because 1 ASPPH member can confer degrees at multiple levels.
[b]The number of schools reporting each year does not sum to the total number of schools because 1 ASPPH member can confer degrees in multiple years.

mixed-effects model (model 2) are presented in Table 3. The adjusted regression models suggested that a 1-percentage-point increase in the proportion of URM residents 20 to 35 years of age in the state population was associated with 0.3-percentage-point increase ($P < .001$) in the proportion of URM graduates among US citizen graduates overall (Table 3, model 1). In addition, a 1-percentage-point increase in the proportion of URM faculty members was associated with a 0.7-percentage-point increase in the proportion of URM graduates ($P < .001$). Conversely, the proportion of graduates who earned their degrees in biostatistics was negatively associated with the proportion of URM graduates ($b = -0.28$; $P < .01$). The proportion of URM graduates with doctoral degrees was 8.9 percentage points less than the proportion with bachelor's degrees ($P < .01$), confirming the trend line shown in Figure 1. We did not find any significant associations between other characteristics and student diversity.

The robustness check with school- or program-level random effects and year fixed effects (Table 3, model 2) confirmed the positive relationship between the proportion of URM graduates among state residents 20 to 35 years of age and the proportion of URM graduates ($b = 0.41$; $P < .001$). Our results remained robust for the associations between faculty diversity and graduate diversity ($b = 0.32$; $P < .01$) and between the proportion of biostatistics graduates and student diversity ($b = -0.19$; $P < .01$).

Subgroup Analyses

The subgroup analysis by degree levels is presented in Table A (available as a supplement to the online version of this article at http://www.ajph.org). The results for bachelor's degree programs revealed a positive relationship between the proportion of URM faculty and graduate diversity ($b = 0.90$; $P < .001$). All other statistically significant relationships from the main models were nonsignificant, but the direction of the effect did not change. We also found that bachelor's degrees provided by public institutions were associated with a 14.5-percentage-point ($P < .01$) higher proportion of URM graduates than bachelors' degrees from private institutions. The findings from the analysis on graduate degree programs were more aligned with the regression results presented in Table 3.

Table B (available as a supplement to the online version of this article at http://www.ajph.org) includes subgroup analyses for Black and Hispanic graduates. The results show statistically significant relationships between the proportion of Black or Hispanic individuals 20 to 35 years of age in the state and the proportion of corresponding

TABLE 2— Summary Diversity Index Statistics for Graduates, Student Body Composition, and Faculty Composition Among ASPPH Member Schools and Programs in the Analytic Sample: United States, 2016–2020

	No.	Mean ±SD	Median (Range)
Percentage of graduates by area of study			
Distance learning	806	9.43 ±20.99	0 (0–100)
Biostatistics	806	4.08 ±7.03	0 (0–45.45)
Epidemiology	806	14.44 ±15.53	10.5 (0–100)
General public health	806	23.24 ±37.36	0 (0–100)
Global health	806	2.99 ±8.90	0 (0–100)
Maternal and child health	806	1.24 ±4.29	0 (0–40.37)
Health policy and management	806	13.75 ±15.39	9.09 (0–81.32)
Percentage of foreign students among grand total	806	10.64 ±10.26	7.69 (0–48.39)
Diversity index			
URM graduates	806	0.78 ±0.47	0.68 (0–4.09)
Black graduates	806	1.07 ±1.12	0.88 (0–12.28)
Hispanic graduates	806	0.59 ±0.49	0.51 (0–3.94)
NH/PI graduates	785	2.26 ±16.52	0 (0–382.89)
AI/AN graduates	805	1.40 ±4.28	0 (0–42.04)
Percentage of FTE faculty by race/ethnicity			
URM	806	14.28 ±10.00	11.69 (0–59.14)
Black	806	8.53 ±8.00	6.35 (0–55.26)
Hispanic	806	5.02 ±5.82	3.42 (0–39.28)
NH/PI	806	0.28 ±1.45	0 (0–16.42)
AI/AN	806	0.45 ±2.88	0 (0–48.39)
Race unknown	806	2.34 ±4.48	0 (0–37.01)

Note. AI/AN = American Indian/Alaska Native; ASPPH = Association of Schools and Programs of Public Health; FTE = full-time equivalent; NH/PI = Native Hawaiian/Pacific Islander; URM = underrepresented minority.

URM graduates (for Black graduates: b = 0.43; $P < .001$; for Hispanic graduates: b = 0.37; $P < .001$).

Master's Degree Program Analysis

Finally, we extended our analysis to include the diversity of the school or program's master's degree applicant pool (Table C, available as a supplement to the online version of this article at http://www.ajph.org). The length of study for master's degree programs is 2 years in general, but to account for the possibility of an extended academic cycle we used 2 measures of applicant diversity: (1) the proportion of URM applicants 2 years in the past and (2) the aggregate number of URM applicants 2 years and 3 years in the past divided by the aggregate total number of domestic applicants 2 years and 3 years in the past.

Overall, our results remained robust. Extended analyses confirmed that the proportion of URM graduates among state residents 20 to 35 years of age (b = 0.13; $P < .01$, b = 0.13; $P = .01$) and the proportion of URM faculty members (b = 0.37; $P < .001$, b = 0.46; $P < .001$) were positively related to the proportion of URM graduates in master's degree programs. In neither analysis did we find a statistically significant relationship between the proportion of graduates who earned a biostatistics degree and the proportion of URM graduates. Most important, we found a positive relationship between the proportion of URM applicants and the proportion of URM graduates (b = 0.73; $P < .001$, b = 0.7; $P < .001$).

DISCUSSION

In this study, we used a unique ASPPH longitudinal data set to examine institutional characteristics associated with the diversity of the association's public health student cohort. To our knowledge, this is the first study to explore the diversity of public health schools and programs by creating an index of diversity at the institutional level. Our findings suggest that although the diversity of the public health educational pipeline has shown an upward trend, racial and ethnic minority graduates continue to remain underrepresented in public health. In addition, we found that several institutional characteristics such as faculty diversity, program degree level, and area of study were associated with the diversity of institutions' public health student cohorts.

In our study, the mean DI score for URM graduates across all degree levels was 0.78, but scores varied by race and ethnicity. For example, although the mean DI scores for Black, Native Hawaiian/Pacific Islander, and American Indian/Alaska Native graduates were greater than 1, the score for Hispanic

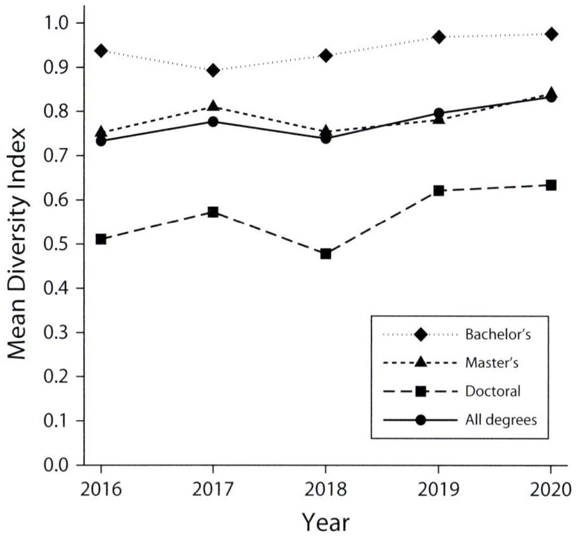

FIGURE 1— Mean Diversity Index Trend Lines for ASPPH Member Schools and Programs in the Analytic Sample: United States, 2016–2020

Note. ASPPH = Association of Schools and Programs of Public Health.

graduates was far less than 1, suggesting that Hispanic students are significantly underrepresented in the public health graduate cohort. As we explored the DI score distribution for each minority group, we found a highly skewed distribution of Native Hawaiian/Pacific Islander and American Indian/Alaska Native graduates, implying that the DI scores for those groups were driven by a few institutions.

Our results regarding the overall lack of diversity in the future public health workforce are consistent with those from a previous study conducted by Goodman et al.[13] However, our findings provide insight into school-level diversity relative to the diversity of the communities in which schools and programs are located. As schools consider strategies to improve the diversity of their student bodies, DI scores provide an overall assessment of areas in which recruitment and retention efforts can be focused. They can also serve as potential tools for accountability and track the diversity of the public health academic pipeline.

Another important finding was that the diversity of applicants to public health programs has improved, but diversity in enrollments continues to lag. We also found that the diversity of the student cohort decreases with higher degree levels, with the highest diversity at the bachelor's degree level. This increased racial/ethnic diversity among students pursuing a bachelor's degree in public health has the potential to subsequently increase diversity among graduate students and, ultimately, faculty and leaders in public health. Racial and ethnic minority students often face systemic barriers to higher education such as financial barriers and lack of early exposure to public health sciences. Public health schools and programs can address these systemic barriers through student-focused initiatives such as information sessions on the application process and financial aid and provision of grants or scholarships and resources for URM students (e.g., pre-entrance summer programs, mentoring programs).[13,20,21]

Given its social justice focus, the public heath discipline can be an attractive career path, particularly for those underrepresented in the sciences and health professions (e.g., individuals from racial and ethnic minority groups, first-generation students, students of low socioeconomic status).[22] In addition, COVID-19 has brought public health to the forefront and generated a renewed interest in the field. According to a recent ASPPH report, public health programs saw a surge in interest between March 2020 and March 2021, with applications to master's in public health programs increasing by 40%.[23]

As public health graduates are an essential part of the educational pipeline that feeds into the public health workforce, this growing interest in public health should be leveraged and mechanisms for recruiting and retaining a diverse workforce should be prioritized. Institutions conferring public health degrees thus play a critical role in improving the diversity of this educational pipeline. As a result, policies to improve the diversity of the workforce will need to focus on diversifying the educational pipeline through complex transformations of the education system. For example, admission processes and decisions need to actively incorporate student-centric approaches such as holistic reviews of applications as opposed to a focus on only grade-point average and standardized test scores.[20,21] Also, recruitment strategies can be intentional in terms of improving the diversity of the public health student cohort, and schools and programs can be held accountable by

TABLE 3— Associations Between State Population Racial Diversity, Institutional Characteristics, and Diversity of Graduates: ASPPH Member Schools and Programs, United States, 2016–2020

	Percentage of URM Graduates, b (95% CI)	
	Model 1: OLS (n = 806)	Model 2: RE + FE (n = 806)
Percentage of URM graduates among state residents aged 20–35 y	0.30 (0.18, 0.41)	0.41 (0.27, 0.55)
Percent of graduates by area of study		
Distance-based program	0.03 (−0.04, 0.11)	0.02 (−0.05, 0.10)
Biostatistics	−0.28 (−0.45, −0.11)	−0.19 (−0.33, −0.05)
Epidemiology	0.05 (−0.06, 0.16)	−0.01 (−0.10, 0.08)
General public health	0.02 (−0.05, 0.09)	0.04 (−0.00, 0.09)
Global health	−0.03 (−0.16, 0.11)	0.13 (0.01, 0.26)
Maternal and child health	−0.05 (−0.28, 0.19)	−0.02 (−0.23, 0.19)
Health policy and management	−0.03 (−0.14, 0.08)	−0.00 (−0.08, 0.07)
Percentage of foreign graduates among grand total	0.16 (−0.01, 0.32)	0.05 (−0.08, 0.17)
Percentage of FTE faculty by race/ethnicity		
URM	0.70 (0.41, 0.99)	0.32 (0.10, 0.55)
Race unknown	0.06 (−0.23, 0.34)	0.07 (−0.20, 0.35)
Degree level (Ref = bachelor's degree)		
Master's degree	−3.65 (−8.08, 0.79)	−1.87 (−5.59, 1.85)
Doctoral degree	−8.91 (−14.47, −3.34)	−4.98 (−10.18, 0.22)
Institution type (Ref = public health program)		
Graduate school of public health	3.18 (−1.16, 7.53)	2.77 (−1.26, 6.81)
Institution ownership type (Ref = private)		
Public	2.40 (−1.47, 6.27)	0.59 (−3.74, 4.92)
Constant	2.52 (−5.64, 10.68)	
Member RE	No	Yes
Year FE	No	Yes

Note. ASPPH = Association of Schools and Programs of Public Health; CI = confidence interval; FE = fixed effect; FTE = full-time equivalent; OLS = ordinary least squares; RE = random effect; URM = underrepresented minority. Standard errors were clustered at the ASPPH member level. The estimated regression coefficient represents percentage-point changes in the percentage of URM graduates associated with 1 percentage point in each explanatory variable.

improving the transparency and availability of their diversity data.[24]

Universities and colleges promulgate "diversity plans" that propose goals for student and faculty diversity, as well as retention plans for maintaining diversity among those groups. Faculty diversity is viewed as important from the perspective of offering students a richer instructor background and providing minority students with model instructors. The minority faculty pipeline, in turn, is dependent on the diversity of the graduate student population, which is connected to the diversity of the bachelor's student population. The positive association between faculty diversity and student diversity in our study likely suggests that schools and programs invested in faculty diversity are also invested in student diversity. It could also suggest that students pay close attention to institutional faculty diversity when making academic decisions. Thus, institutions of higher education need to continue to make active investments and push efforts in the recruitment and retention of diverse faculties.[13]

Limitations

Our study involved some limitations. First, because of issues regarding data availability, our conceptualization of diversity was limited to race/ethnicity. Our findings are a starting point to assess the diversity of public health educational institutions. A holistic conceptualization of diversity in the future could consider the intersectionality of critical factors such as income and class with race/ethnicity. This could better predict what drives student diversity and highlight systemic root causes (e.g., poverty, lack of resources) that stymie diversity.

Second, our analysis included only schools and programs of public health that are ASPPH members. Although this limits the external validity of our findings, our methods can be extrapolated to measure diversity at schools and programs that are not ASPPH members. Third, because of the lack of data, we combined racial and ethnic minority groups. To achieve the goal of health equity, better access to granular data on race/ethnicity and other drivers of diversity such as income or class and being a first-generation student is critical to track the diversity of the public health workforce. Accreditation bodies can incentivize institutions of higher education to collect such data.

Fourth, our data were reported by ASPPH members and may be subject to nonresponse error. Finally, in the DI, the population of the state in which a school or program was located was used as the denominator. It is likely that some institutions (such as privately owned schools and programs) have higher proportions of students who are from outside their region. However, because a majority of the schools and programs included in our study were publicly owned, we used the state population as the denominator. Future research can explore constructing diversity indexes with different denominators and weighting strategies.

Public Health Implications

We have identified opportunities for public health schools and programs to reflect on their role in contributing to a diverse public health workforce. A diverse student body is integral to the higher education experience in the United States given that students gain education not only in the classroom but also by interacting with a wide spectrum of fellow students. In addition, providing access to higher education improves social mobility among students who have historically not had access to the opportunities that education creates. The $7.7 billion devoted to expanding the public health workforce under the American Rescue Plan Act of 2021 is a window of opportunity to make significant investments in improving the diversity of our public health workforce.[24]

Data-driven strategies are necessary for enhancing workforce diversity. However, workforce data, and more specifically diversity-related data, are not regularly tracked nationally. To that end, our study's findings engender transparency through an evidence-driven analysis of the current state of public health education.[24] AJPH

ABOUT THE AUTHORS

Anushree Vichare and Yoon Hong Park are with the Fitzhugh Mullan Institute for Health Workforce Equity and the Department of Health Policy and Management, Milken Institute School of Public Health, George Washington University, Washington, DC. Christine M. Plepys is with the Association of Schools and Programs of Public Health, Washington, DC.

CORRESPONDENCE

Correspondence should be sent to Anushree Vichare, PhD, MPH, MBBS, 950 New Hampshire Ave, Suite #603, Washington, DC 20052 (e-mail: avichare@gwu.edu). Reprints can be ordered at http://www.ajph.org by clicking the "Reprints" link.

PUBLICATION INFORMATION

Full Citation: Vichare A, Park YH, Plepys CM. Diversity of the US public health workforce pipeline (2016–2020): role of academic institutions. *Am J Public Health*. 2023;113(9): 1000–1008.

Acceptance Date: May 20, 2023.

DOI: https://doi.org/10.2105/AJPH.2023.307352

CONTRIBUTORS

A. Vichare conceptualized and designed the study, acquired data, interpreted the results, and drafted the initial version of the article. Y. H. Park analyzed the data, interpreted the results, and assisted with the drafting of the initial version of the article. C. M. Plepys provided the study data, advised on study conceptualization and study design, and provided feedback on subsequent drafts of the article.

ACKNOWLEDGMENTS

This research was supported by the Bureau of Health Workforce, National Center for Health Workforce Analysis, Health Resources and Services Administration (HRSA), US Department of Health and Human Services (DHHS) as part of an award totaling $450,000.

We are grateful to Edward Salsberg and Erin Brantley for their support in the conceptualization of the study and the adaptation of the diversity index.

Note. The contents are those of the authors and do not necessarily represent the official views of or an endorsement by the HRSA, the DHHS, or the US government.

CONFLICTS OF INTEREST

The authors have no conflicts of interest to disclose.

HUMAN PARTICIPANT PROTECTION

This study involved data aggregated at the public health school/program level and did not include human participants. Thus, the study was exempt from institutional review board and informed consent requirements.

REFERENCES

1. Moore JT, Ricaldi JN, Rose CE, et al. Disparities in incidence of COVID-19 among underrepresented racial/ethnic groups in counties identified as hotspots during June 5–18, 2020—22 States, February–June 2020. *MMWR Morb Mortal Wkly Rep*. 2020;69(33):1122–1126. https://doi.org/10.15585/mmwr.mm6933e1
2. Karmakar M, Lantz PM, Tipirneni R. Association of social and demographic factors with COVID-19 incidence and death rates in the US. *JAMA Netw Open*. 2021;4(1):e2036462. https://doi.org/10.1001/jamanetworkopen.2020.36462
3. Mitchell DA, Lassiter SL. Addressing health care disparities and increasing workforce diversity: the next step for the dental, medical, and public health professions. *Am J Public Health*. 2006; 96(12):2093–2097. https://doi.org/10.2105/AJPH.2005.082818
4. Cohen JJ, Gabriel BA, Terrell C. The case for diversity in the health care workforce. *Health Aff (Millwood)*. 2017;21(5):90–102. https://doi.org/10.1377/HLTHAFF.21.5.90
5. Jackson CS, Nadine Gracia J. Addressing health and health-care disparities: the role of a diverse workforce and the social determinants of health. *Public Health Rep*. 2014;129(suppl 2):57–61. https://doi.org/10.1177/00333549141291S211
6. Saha S, Shipman SA. Race-neutral versus race-conscious workforce policy to improve access to care. *Health Aff (Millwood)*. 2008;27(1):234–245. https://doi.org/10.1377/hlthaff.27.1.234
7. Sellers K, Leider JP, Gould E, et al. The state of the US governmental public health workforce, 2014–2017. *Am J Public Health*. 2019;109(5): 674–680. https://doi.org/10.2105/AJPH.2019.305011
8. Bogaert K, Castrucci BC, Gould E, et al. The Public Health Workforce Interests and Needs Survey (PH WINS 2017): an expanded perspective on the state health agency workforce. *J Public Health Manag Pract*. 2019;25(2):S16–S25. https://doi.org/10.1097/PHH.0000000000000932
9. Juliano C, Castrucci BC, Leider JP, McGinty MD, Bogaert K. The governmental public health workforce in 26 cities: PH WINS results from Big Cities Health Coalition members. *J Public Health Manag Pract*. 2019;25(2):S38–S48. https://doi.org/10.1097/PHH.0000000000000929
10. Leider JP, Plepys CM, Castrucci BC, Burke EM, Blakely CH. Trends in the conferral of graduate public health degrees: a triangulated approach. *Public Health Rep*. 2018;133(6):729–737. https://doi.org/10.1177/0033354918791542

11. Leider JP, Castrucci BC, Plepys CM, Blakely C, Burke E, Sprague JB. Characterizing the growth of the undergraduate public health major: US, 1992–2012. *Public Health Rep.* 2015;130(1):104–113. https://doi.org/10.1177/003335491513000114
12. Healton CG. The shape of our river. *Am J Prev Med.* 1999;16(suppl 3):1–4. https://doi.org/10.1016/S0749-3797(99)00047-1
13. Goodman MS, Plepys CM, Bather JR, Kelliher RM, Healton CG. Racial/ethnic diversity in academic public health: 20-year update. *Public Health Rep.* 2020;135(1):74–81. https://doi.org/10.1177/0033354919887747
14. Franklin RS. The roles of population, place, and institution in student diversity in American higher education. *Growth Change.* 2013;44(1):30–53. https://doi.org/10.1111/grow.12001
15. Franklin RS. Benchmarking student diversity at public universities in the United States: accounting for state population composition. *Ann Reg Sci.* 2012;49(2):355–372. https://doi.org/10.1007/s00168-011-0454-4
16. Salsberg E, Richwine C, Westergaard S, et al. Estimation and comparison of current and future racial/ethnic representation in the US health care workforce. *JAMA Netw Open.* 2021;4(3):e213789. https://doi.org/10.1001/jamanetworkopen.2021.3789
17. Leider JP, Castrucci BC, Robins M, et al. The exodus of state and local public health employees: separations started before and continued throughout COVID-19. *Health Aff (Millwood).* 2023;42(3):338–348. https://doi.org/10.1377/hlthaff.2022.01251
18. National Science Foundation. Women, minorities, and persons with disabilities in science and engineering: 2019. Available at: https://ncses.nsf.gov/pubs/nsf19304/digest. Accessed April 11, 2023.
19. Kreuter MW, Griffith DJ, Thompson V, et al. Lessons learned from a decade of focused recruitment and training to develop minority public health professionals. *Public Health.* 2011;101:188–195. https://doi.org/10.2105/AJPH.2011.300122
20. Duffus WA, Trawick C, Moonesinghe R, Tola J, Truman BI, Dean HD. Training racial and ethnic minority students for careers in public health sciences. *Am J Prev Med.* 2014;47(suppl 3):S368–S375. https://doi.org/10.1016/j.amepre.2014.07.028
21. Sullivan LW. Missing persons: minorities in the health professions. Available at: https://campaignforaction.org/wp-content/uploads/2016/04/SullivanReport-Diversity-in-Healthcare-Workforce1.pdf. Accessed August 7, 2022.
22. Fernandez M. The Fauci effect: interest spikes in health crisis communication. Available at: https://www.axios.com/2021/05/27/the-fauci-effect-interest-spikes-in-health-crisis-communication. Accessed August 4, 2022.
23. Coronado F, Beck AJ, Shah G, Young JL, Sellers K, Leider JP. Understanding the dynamics of diversity in the public health workforce. *J Public Health Manag Pract.* 2020;26(4):389–392. https://doi.org/10.1097/PHH.0000000000001075
24. American Rescue Plan Act of 2021. Available at: https://www.congress.gov/bill/117th-congress/house-bill/1319/text. Accessed August 7, 2022.

Self-Reported Barriers to Care Among Sexual and Gender Minority People With Disabilities: Findings From The PRIDE Study, 2019–2020

Shane Lamba, MPH, Juno Obedin-Maliver, MD, MPH, MAS, Jonathan Mayo, MPH, Annesa Flentje, PhD, Micah E. Lubensky, PhD, Zubin Dastur, MS, MPH, and Mitchell R. Lunn, MD, MAS

Objectives. To examine the associations of self-reported disability status with health care access barriers for sexual and gender minority (SGM) people.

Methods. The Population Research in Identity and Disparities for Equality (PRIDE) Study participants lived in the United States or its territories, completed the 2019 annual questionnaire (n = 4961), and self-reported their disability and health care access experiences, including whether they had a primary care provider, were uninsured, delayed care, and were unable to obtain care. We classified disabilities as physical, mental, intellectual, and other; compared participants to those without disabilities; and performed logistic regression to determine the associations of disability status and health care access barriers.

Results. SGM people with disabilities were less likely to have a usual place to seek health care (69.0% vs 75.3%; $P \leq .001$) and more often reported being mistreated or disrespected as reasons to delay care (29.0% vs 10.2%; $P \leq .001$). SGM people with disabilities were more likely to delay care (adjusted odds ratio [AOR] = 3.28; 95% confidence interval [CI] = 2.83, 3.81) and be unable to obtain care (AOR = 3.10; 95% CI = 2.59, 3.71).

Conclusions. Future work should address culturally competent health care to ameliorate disparities for the SGM disability community. (*Am J Public Health*. 2023;113(9):1009–1018. https://doi.org/10.2105/AJPH.2023.307333)

AJPH September 2023, Vol 113, No. 9

According to the Centers for Disease Control and Prevention (CDC), an estimated 61 million adults (~26%) in the United States live with a disability, and approximately 33% of people with disabilities do not have a regular health care provider.[1,2] Racial and ethnic minority groups (e.g., Blacks/African Americans, Hispanics/Latinos, Native Americans), women, and older adults are at an increased risk of living with a disability over their lifetime.[1,2] Documented health disparities for people with disabilities include poorer access to health care services, experiences of discrimination, lower health insurance rates, poorer access to medications, and delaying or being unable to obtain care compared with people without disabilities.[3–6] Additionally, people with disabilities are disproportionately from lower socioeconomic status groups, which has been shown to affect health care utilization rates, especially because of the inability to pay for health care services.[4,5]

Although there are documented disparities in health care access for people with disabilities, few studies have explored differences in health care access, such as having a usual place to seek care and having a primary care provider (PCP), for sexual and gender minority (SGM) people with disabilities. SGM people face numerous challenges when seeking health care, and access to knowledgeable practitioners is limited; therefore, the health care needs of SGM people are often overlooked. SGM communities report harassment, disrespect, and discrimination, because of which delays in care occur, reducing the likelihood of receiving needed screening tests (e.g., cisgender lesbian women and transgender men were less likely to complete regular cervical cancer screening than are cisgender heterosexual patients).[7–9]

SGM women, for example, had delayed breast cancer diagnoses and faster recurrence than did cisgender heterosexual women.[10] Transgender people are 5 times more likely to report poor quality of care with regard to routine visits, and (presumably cisgender) lesbian, gay, or bisexual (LGB) people are 2 times more likely to delay care than are non-LGB people.[11] It is evident, as we noted, that there are barriers to care; unfortunately, there is limited research about the multiplicative barriers present for SGM people living with disabilities. We expect that the overarching barriers and unmet needs in SGM communities are also present in the SGM disability community.

SGM people have been historically invisible in national, state, and local public health surveillance systems through exclusion of comprehensive sexual orientation and gender identity questions.[12] Without these questions, pervasive SGM health gaps remain—especially for SGM people with disabilities. SGM people with disabilities have experienced homonegative (also known as "heterosexism") and ableist microaggressions that are greatly associated with mental health conditions such as depression.[13] Additionally, SGM cisgender women with disabilities face more discrimination and higher rates of posttraumatic stress disorder, feelings of anxiety, and lack of connectedness with the lesbian, gay, bisexual, and transgender (LGBT) community than do SGM cisgender women without disabilities. They also report poor quality of life related to their physical health.[14]

Consequently, several goals of Healthy People 2030 involve promoting steady access to health care services and decreasing barriers to care for people with disabilities and the lesbian, gay, bisexual, transgender, and queer (LGBTQ+) or SGM communities.[15,16] However, current research shows that both people with disabilities and SGM people face barriers when seeking health care. SGM people with disabilities, an even more marginalized group, may encounter multiple risks and barriers to accessing care. We address the existing gap in knowledge by examining the differences in health care access between SGM people with and without disabilities.

METHODS

The Population Research in Identity and Disparities for Equality (PRIDE) Study is an online, national, community-engaged, prospective cohort study of SGM adults in the United States. Details about The PRIDE Study, including eligibility criteria, are reported elsewhere.[17] We recruited participants via convenience sampling through PRIDEnet—a national network of organizations that engage with SGM communities—digital communications, word of mouth, and outreach at conferences and events.

To be included in this analysis, participants must have answered the question "Do you currently identify as a person with a disability?" Response options were binary (yes vs no). We categorized participants into 2 cohorts: SGM people with any disability and SGM people with no disability. We asked participants, "What condition(s) or problem(s) are related to your disability identity?" We classified SGM people with disabilities into 4 distinct disability categories, employing the CDC's classification of disability as a framework: physical (e.g., cancer, circulatory diseases, paralysis), mental (e.g., anxiety, depression, memory issues), intellectual and developmental (e.g., attention deficit disorder, autism, learning disabilities), and other.[18]

This definition of disability focuses on any condition of the body or mind that makes it harder for the person to do activities and interact with the world around them.[18] Details on the disabilities in each category can be found in Appendix A (available as a supplement to the online version of this article at http://www.ajph.org). The disability type categorization was not mutually exclusive; participants could select multiple disability categories and did not choose a primary diagnosis. There were 337 free-text disabilities that 2 authors (S. L., M. R. L.) classified into the 4 categories. The free-text disabilities in Appendix A, Table A, are verbatim and unedited; there are redundancies and misspellings.

Sociodemographic Characteristics

We collected the data used in this study in The PRIDE Study's 2019 Annual Questionnaire between July 1, 2019, and May 28, 2020, which we administered via Qualtrics (Qualtrics, LLC, Provo, UT) on the study's Web-based research platform.[17] We tabulated sociodemographic characteristics, such as age, sexual orientation, gender identity, income level, and race/ethnicity. Regarding sexual orientation, we asked participants, "What is your current sexual orientation?" and regarding gender identity, we asked participants, "What is your current gender identity?" Participants could select all relevant categories.

Health Care Access

Health care access variables included questions about whether the participant had a PCP, whether they had a usual place of care, what type of health care facility they utilized, and whether they had access to transgender-related health care. We took all the health care access measures from the National Health Interview Survey, excluding questions specific to transgender people.[19]

We asked participants, "Is there a place that you usually go to when you are sick or need advice about your health?" with answer choices of "Yes," "No," "There is no place," "There is more than one place," and "I don't know." We asked participants who answered the preceding question with "Yes" or "There is more than one place," "Is that the same place you usually go when you need routine or preventive care, such as a physical examination or checkup?"

Additional questions we asked all participants included "Do you have a PCP?", "Have you seen your PCP in the past 12 months?", and "In the past 12 months, was there any time when you did not have any health insurance or coverage?" with response options of "Yes," "No," and "I don't know." We also asked them, "During the past 12 months, did you have any trouble finding a general doctor or health care provider who would see you?" with response options of "Yes," "No," "I haven't tried," and "I don't know." We asked participants who identified as either a gender minority or both a gender and sexual minority the following: "In the past 12 months, have you gone to a doctor, health care provider or clinic for transgender-related health care?" and "Does the person or place who provides your transgender-related health care also take care of your overall general health?" Response choices for both questions were "Yes," "No," and "I don't know."

Delaying Care

The variables related to delaying care included being denied or given lower quality of care; being unable to access specific tests, medical care, or treatments; being mistreated or disrespected by health care providers; and being denied or given lower quality mental health care. The delay care measures are from the National Health Interview Survey.[19]

We asked participants the following questions, which had "Yes" or "No" as answer choices: "In the past 12 months, were you delayed in getting medical care, tests, or treatments that you or a health care provider believed necessary?", "In the past 12 months, were you unable to obtain medical care, tests, or treatments that you or a health care provider believed necessary?", "In the past 12 months, have you been denied or given lower quality medical care?", "Was there a time in the past 12 months when you needed to see a health care provider but did not because you thought you would be disrespected or mistreated?", and "In the past 12 months, have you been denied or given lower quality mental health care?"

Data Analysis

We performed analyses in SAS version 9.4 (SAS Institute, Cary, NC). We assessed descriptive statistics for sociodemographic characteristics by disability status: any versus none. We assessed the frequency of categorical variables in the health care access and delaying care domains as count and percentage and compared them by using the χ^2 test. For these comparisons, we included the response option of "I don't know" in the denominators, but we omitted missing data.

To understand the association with disability status and experiencing health care access barriers, we ran separate logistic regression models by disability type (physical, mental, intellectual or developmental, other, and any disability). The outcome variables were (1) having a PCP, (2) delaying care in the past 12 months, (3) being uninsured in the past 12 months, and (4) being unable to obtain care in the past 12 months. We excluded participants from analyses when "I don't know" or the outcome response was missing. SGM people without disabilities were the referent group. We used crude and adjusted logistic regression models and presented associations as odds ratios (ORs) and 95% confidence intervals (CIs). Covariates included in adjusted models were age,[1,2,4] race/ethnicity,[4–7,10] income,[1,3,6] employment status,[6] and education.[7]

We conducted sensitivity analyses to assess the effects of rural versus urban status and noncisgender identity in the logistic regression models. For rural versus urban status, we used the US Department of Agriculture (USDA)–provided crosswalk from participant-provided zip code to USDA rural–urban commuting area code (1–10; 10 = most rural) as a continuous variable.[20]

We assessed whether noncisgender or cisgender status was associated with experiencing health care barriers; further information can be found in Appendix B, Tables A and B (available as a supplement to the online version of this article at http://www.ajph.org).

RESULTS

We included 4961 participants in our study, of whom 1540 (~31%) self-reported a disability. We found significant differences between people with and those without disabilities for age, race/ethnicity, sexual orientation, gender identity, income status, and education levels (each $P \le .001$). The median age for SGM persons with disabilities was slightly younger than those without disabilities (29.8 years [interquartile range (IQR) = 17.1] vs 32.1 years [IQR = 17.6]). SGM persons with disabilities were less likely to be employed than were those without disabilities (61% vs 81%; Table 1).

Health Care Access and Delaying Care

Compared with SGM persons without disabilities, those with disabilities were less likely to have a usual place to seek health care (69% vs 75%; $P \le .001$) and more frequently reported being mistreated or disrespected as reasons to delay care (29% vs 10%; $P \le .001$). There were no significant differences between disability status and having a PCP ($P = .31$), but those with disabilities were more likely to have seen their PCP in the past 12 months ($P = .02$; Table 2).

SGM persons with were more likely than were those without disabilities to have trouble finding a health care provider (18% vs 9%; $P \le .001$), and, among gender minority participants, to not

TABLE 1— Sociodemographic Characteristics of Sexual and Gender Minority Adults in The PRIDE Study by Disability Status: United States, 2019–2020

Sociodemographic Characteristics	Any Disability (n = 1540)	No Disability (n = 3421)
Age, y, median (IQR)	29.8 (17.1)	32.1 (17.6)
Gender identity,[a] no. (%)		
Agender only	14 (0.9)	15 (0.4)
Cisgender man only	82 (5.3)	479 (14.0)
Cisgender woman only	201 (13.0)	670 (19.6)
Genderqueer only	28 (1.8)	34 (1.0)
Man only	100 (6.5)	375 (11.0)
Nonbinary only	102 (6.6)	121 (3.5)
Questioning only	7 (0.5)	7 (0.2)
Transgender man only	67 (4.4)	136 (4.0)
Transgender woman only	40 (2.6)	72 (2.1)
Two-spirit only	1 (0.06)	0 (0.0)
Woman only	90 (5.8)	237 (7.0)
Another gender identity only	15 (1.0)	12 (0.4)
Multiple selections	793 (51.5)	1263 (36.9)
Noncisgender status		
Cisgender	450 (29.6)	1720 (50.7)
Noncisgender	1073 (70.4)	1672 (49.3)
Missing	17	29
Sexual orientation,[a] no. (%)		
Asexual only	40 (2.6)	80 (2.3)
Bisexual only	134 (8.7)	350 (10.3)
Gay only	200 (13.0)	859 (25.2)
Lesbian only	125 (8.1)	409 (12.0)
Pansexual only	55 (3.6)	86 (2.5)
Queer only	133 (8.7)	249 (7.3)
Questioning only	9 (0.6)	6 (0.2)
Same-gender loving only	0 (0.0)	5 (0.2)
Straight only	14 (0.9)	30 (0.9)
Two-spirit only	2 (0.1)	0 (0.0)
Another sexual orientation only	10 (0.7)	11 (0.3)
Multiple selections	815 (53.0)	1331 (39.0)
Missing	3	5
Income, $, no. (%)		
0	178 (11.8)	185 (5.5)
1–20 000	631 (41.7)	775 (23.1)
20 001–40 000	307 (20.3)	702 (21.0)
40 001–60 000	199 (13.1)	554 (16.5)
60 001–80 000	89 (5.9)	385 (11.5)
80 001–100 000	38 (2.5)	240 (7.2)
≥ 100 001	72 (4.7)	515 (15.2)
Missing	26	65

Continued

TABLE 1— Continued

Sociodemographic Characteristics	Any Disability (n = 1540)	No Disability (n = 3421)
Education, no. (%)		
High school or less	141 (9.2)	191 (5.7)
Some college	403 (26.4)	491 (14.5)
2-y college degree	87 (5.7)	115 (3.4)
4-y college degree	492 (32.2)	1185 (34.9)
Graduate school or higher	405 (26.5)	1410 (41.5)
Missing	12	29
Race/ethnicity,[a] no. (%)		
American Indian or Alaska Native only	7 (0.5)	7 (0.2)
Asian only	23 (1.5)	97 (2.9)
Black/African American only	32 (2.1)	64 (1.9)
Hispanic only	28 (1.8)	84 (2.5)
Middle Eastern or North African only	3 (0.2)	12 (0.4)
Native Hawaiian or other Pacific Islander only	0 (0.0)	0 (0.0)
White only	1205 (79.1)	2786 (82.9)
Another race only	12 (0.8)	11 (0.3)
Multiple selections	212 (13.9)	300 (8.9)
Missing	18	60
Employment status, no. (%)		
No	604 (39.5)	635 (18.7)
Yes	925 (60.5)	2758 (81.3)
Missing	11	28
US Census region, no. (%)		
Northeast (region 1)	293 (19.2)	704 (20.8)
Midwest (region 2)	335 (22.0)	660 (19.5)
South (region 3)	396 (26.0)	886 (26.1)
West (region 4)	501 (32.9)	1132 (33.4)
Other (US possessions, military overseas)	0 (0.0)	9 (0.3)
RUCA, no. (%)		
RUCA 1–3 (metropolitan)	1415 (93.0)	3144 (93.1)
RUCA 4–6 (micropolitan)	68 (4.5)	161 (4.8)
RUCA 7–9 (small town)	24 (1.6)	36 (1.1)
RUCA 10 (rural)	15 (1.0)	35 (1.0)
Missing	18	45

Note. IQR = interquartile range; RUCA = rural–urban commuting area. All $P \le .001$, except US Census region $P = .07$ and RUCA $P = .48$.

[a]Gender identity, sexual orientation, and race/ethnicity questions allowed multiple selections.

have gone to a transgender-related health care provider or clinic (51% vs 45%; $P = .02$; Table 3). SGM persons with disabilities were more likely to be denied or given lower quality medical care (22% vs 6%) and were more likely to be denied or given lower quality mental health care (15% vs 4%) than were those without disabilities (each $P \le .001$; Table 3).

Health Care Barriers

SGM persons with physical disabilities (adjusted odds ratio [AOR] = 1.56; 95% CI = 1.23, 1.98) and mental disabilities (AOR = 1.31; 95% CI = 1.08, 1.60) were more likely to have a PCP than were those without disabilities. SGM people with physical (AOR = 4.32; 95% CI = 3.63, 5.15), mental (AOR = 3.61; 95% CI = 3.08, 4.23), intellectual (AOR = 2.86; 95% CI = 2.32, 3.52), and other (AOR = 7.84; 95% CI = 4.99, 12.31) disabilities were more likely to delay care than were those without disabilities. SGM people with physical (AOR = 4.06; 95% CI = 3.31, 4.98), mental (AOR = 3.43; 95% CI = 2.84, 4.14), intellectual (AOR = 3.25; 95% CI = 2.55, 4.14), and other (AOR = 6.45; 95% CI = 4.05, 10.29) disabilities were more likely to be unable to obtain care than were those without disabilities (Table 4). We saw no difference in insurance coverage after adjusting for age, race/ethnicity, income, employment status, and education among all disability groups.

When examining rural–urban commuting area code and noncisgender versus cisgender status as covariates, sensitivity analyses revealed minor AOR changes with no changes to significant findings (Appendix B, Tables B and C).

DISCUSSION

To our knowledge, this is the first study to examine health care access and associated barriers for SGM persons with disabilities. We found that SGM persons with disabilities experienced significant barriers to health care access, including delaying care because of mistreatment or disrespect, being denied or given lower quality medical care, being uninsured, and not having a usual place of care. These findings show the need to

TABLE 2— Differences With Health Care Access Measures for Sexual and Gender Minority People in The PRIDE Study by Disability Status: United States, 2019–2020

	Any Disability (n = 1540), No. (%)	No Disability (n = 3421), No. (%)
Has usual place of care		
No	125 (8.53)	302 (9.22)
Yes	1012 (69.08)	2468 (75.31)
More than 1	294 (20.07)	430 (13.12)
I don't know	34 (2.32)	77 (2.35)
Missing	75	144
Has routine place of care		
No	137 (10.55)	262 (9.07)
Yes	1147 (88.37)	2609 (90.31)
I don't know	14 (1.08)	18 (0.62)
Missing	8	9
Not applicable	234	523
Trouble finding health care provider in past 12 mo		
No	1107 (75.51)	2758 (84.32)
Yes	268 (18.28)	277 (8.47)
I haven't tried	72 (4.91)	220 (6.73)
I don't know	19 (1.30)	16 (0.49)
Missing	74	150
Has a PCP		
No	219 (14.93)	535 (16.36)
Yes	1216 (82.89)	2678 (81.87)
I don't know	32	58
Seen PCP in past 12 mo[a]		
No	85 (7.10)	323 (12.19)
Yes	1104 (92.23)	2312 (87.28)
I don't know	8	14
Uninsured in past 12 mo		
No	1232 (84.04)	2864 (87.48)
Yes	212 (14.46)	393 (12.00)
I don't know	22 (1.50)	17 (0.52)
Sought transgender-related health care in past 12 mo[b]		
No	414 (50.86)	447 (44.7)
Yes	395 (48.53)	550 (55.00)
I don't know	5 (0.61)	3 (0.30)
Transgender-related health care also takes care of your general health[c]		
No	157 (39.75)	221 (40.26)
Yes	233 (58.99)	319 (58.11)
I don't know	5 (1.27)	9 (1.64)

Note. PCP = primary care provider.

[a]Participants were asked this question if they had a PCP.
[b]Only gender minority or both sexual minority and gender minority participants were asked this question.
[c]Only gender minority or both sexual minority and gender minority participants that sought transgender-related care in the past 12 mo were asked this question.

gather more data to fully understand health care utilization in this specific population, and they provide an understanding of the current state of health care–related barriers for the SGM community. Many of our findings in this study were also presented in previous work exploring the quality of health care for the SGM community (regardless of disability status), including lack of culturally competent care,[7,8,21–23] structural and systemic barriers to adequate collection of sexual orientation and gender identity,[22,23] and poor provider education for comprehensive SGM health care.[11,21,22,24] Therefore, our study serves as a call to action for public health systems and practitioners to reduce the barriers this population experiences.

Nearly one third of participants indicated that they had a disability, which is higher than the general population estimate of approximately 25%.[2,6,25] Prevalence data are essential to understanding the rates at which disability occurs in the SGM community. It was unclear why disability status was higher in our cohort; a possible explanation is that SGM people have complex health histories or conditions,[26,27] further exposing SGM people to more disabling health. Future studies should collect information regarding the onset of disability and why disability has developed among these individuals. Nonetheless, more research should be implemented to better appreciate the breadth of factors affecting disability status, such as social, cultural, and medical.

Implications of Delaying Care

We have reported alarming differences in the rates of delaying care for SGM people with versus those without

TABLE 3— Differences With Delaying Care Among Sexual and Gender Minority People With Any Disability and No Disability in The PRIDE Study: United States, 2019–2020

Delay Care Measures	Any Disability (n = 1540), No. (%)	No Disability (n = 3421), No. (%)
Delayed medical care in past 12 mo		
No	866 (59.03)	2746 (84.10)
Yes	601 (40.97)	519 (15.90)
Not applicable/missing	73	156
Unable to obtain medical care in past 12 mo		
No	1092 (74.54)	2993 (91.50)
Yes	373 (25.46)	278 (8.50)
Not applicable/missing	75	150
Denied or given lower quality care in past 12 mo		
No	1155 (78.20)	3070 (94.03)
Yes	322 (21.80)	195 (5.97)
Not applicable/missing	63	156
Delayed care because of disrespect or mistreatment in past 12 mo		
No	1073 (70.97)	3024 (89.81)
Yes	439 (29.03)	343 (10.19)
Not applicable/missing	28	54
Denied or given lower quality mental health care in past 12 mo		
No	1096 (84.83)	2483 (95.79)
Yes	196 (15.17)	109 (4.21)
Not applicable/missing	248	829

disabilities. SGM people with disabilities had up to 8 times greater odds of delaying care in the past 12 months. These were 1 to 3 times higher than in studies on non-SGM people with disabilities.[3–5,28,29] The top reasons for delaying care were the costs associated with care, poor insurance coverage, and lack of appointments. Our findings support previous work that noted similar barriers of affordability, insurance coverage, and lack of appointments as drivers to delaying care.[3,4,28,30,31] We observed that people with disabilities had lower socioeconomic status (e.g., levels of income and education) and higher rates of unemployment. This may explain the greater financial barriers to health care access, which are known to influence accessing care.[32,33]

Transportation issues and physical limitations owing to disability were also stated as barriers in the literature.[3,4,28,30,31] To minimize these barriers, telemedicine could be adopted to improve access with LGBTQ+-affirming providers.[34] Although we did not find significant differences after adjusting for rural status, rural status may exacerbate barriers associated with accessing care; future work should explore the role it may play among multiple marginalized communities.[33,35] Our data can equip public health practitioners to prioritize future health policies to decrease care costs and increase appointment availability, which would notably increase access for all people with disabilities.[36]

Negative Health Care Experiences

In addition to socioeconomic and health care access barriers, disrespect and mistreatment were 2 reasons that people delayed care. SGM people with disabilities were approximately 3 times more likely to delay care because of disrespect or mistreatment than were those without disabilities. Existing studies reported disproportionate experiences with discrimination, mistreatment, stigma, and bias among SGM people seeking health care.[7,21,37] Moreover, SGM people with disabilities feared being discriminated against in health care settings and not being understood because of their multiple identities.[38] The participants' responses included hesitation interacting with health care providers, lack of wellness services, and poorly trained (or incompetent) health care systems. Combining previous studies' findings with this study's findings leads to the conclusion that cultural sensitivity and competency trainings for health care providers and systems may be necessary to mitigate SGM people with disabilities' decisions to delay care.

Furthermore, SGM people with disabilities had 3 to 6 times higher odds of being unable to obtain care than did SGM people without disabilities. This finding was compelling because a higher proportion of those with disabilities had a PCP, which we assumed would increase their ability to obtain care. However, having a PCP did not improve access to care issues. Many reasons for being unable to obtain care were similar to the reasons for delaying care, including costs, insurance coverage, and appointment availability. Nevertheless, this reinforces the need to address the barriers with policy

TABLE 4— Odds Ratios of Disability Type in Relation to Experiencing Health Care Barriers for Sexual and Gender Minority People in The PRIDE Study: United States, 2019–2020

Health Care Barriers	No.	COR (95% CI)	AOR (95% CI)
Having a PCP			
No disability	2678	1 (Ref)	1 (Ref)
Physical	778	1.47 (1.17, 1.83)	1.56 (1.23, 1.98)
Mental	967	1.04 (0.87, 1.25)	1.31 (1.08, 1.60)
Intellectual	419	0.95 (0.74, 1.22)	1.27 (0.98, 1.65)
Other	78	1.30 (0.70, 2.40)	1.36 (0.72, 2.57)
Any disability	1216	1.11 (0.93, 1.32)	1.32 (1.10, 1.59)
Being uninsured in past 12 mo			
No disability	393	1 (Ref)	1 (Ref)
Physical	124	1.19 (0.96, 1.48)	0.93 (0.74, 1.18)
Mental	185	1.38 (1.14, 1.67)	1.03 (0.84, 1.26)
Intellectual	80	1.35 (1.04, 1.75)	0.96 (0.73, 1.26)
Other	14	1.33 (0.74, 2.36)	1.01 (0.55, 1.87)
Any disability	212	1.25 (1.05, 1.50)	0.96 (0.79, 1.17)
Delaying care in past 12 mo			
No disability	519	1 (Ref)	1 (Ref)
Physical	412	4.49 (3.82, 5.28)	4.32 (3.63, 5.15)
Mental	520	4.18 (3.60, 4.85)	3.61 (3.08, 4.23)
Intellectual	208	3.49 (2.86, 4.26)	2.86 (2.32, 3.52)
Other	56	8.23 (5.36, 12.64)	7.84 (4.99, 12.31)
Any disability	601	3.67 (3.19, 4.22)	3.28 (2.83, 3.81)
Unable to obtain care in past 12 mo			
No disability	278	1 (Ref)	1 (Ref)
Physical	266	4.56 (3.78, 5.51)	4.06 (3.31, 4.98)
Mental	328	4.15 (3.48, 4.95)	3.43 (2.84, 4.14)
Intellectual	143	4.05 (3.22, 5.09)	3.25 (2.55, 4.14)
Other	37	7.38 (4.77, 11.41)	6.45 (4.05, 10.29)
Any disability	373	3.68 (3.10, 4.36)	3.10 (2.59, 3.71)

Note. AOR = adjusted odds ratio; CI = confidence interval; COR = crude odds ratio; PCP = primary care provider.

changes that focus on affordability and expanding access.

Unfortunately, disability status was associated with trouble finding a usual health care provider. Although we did not assess the reasons, a qualitative study explored the breadth of the barriers faced by people with disabilities when accessing health care services.[33] The authors found that people with disabilities were frustrated with trying to understand their insurance coverage and to navigate the limited provider network lists. For these reasons, participants were delaying their care and were unable to find providers that met their needs.[33] Additionally, the participants were concerned about high costs and distances associated with visiting their providers, which made it cumbersome to both afford and receive timely care.[33] These barriers are potentially shared among all people with disabilities, including those identifying as a SGM. Several policy-level implications, such as lowering deductibles, increasing provider network groups, and offering transportation stipends for appointments in health insurance plans, may be necessary to shrink the disparities experienced.

Lastly, we found associations between disability status and being uninsured (14.5% vs 12.0%, respectively $P \le .001$). Compared with population-based studies,[6,28,32] variation exists in the uninsurance rates among people with disabilities (range = 13%–21%). These studies neglected to collect sexual orientation and gender identity information. However, a recent government report noted that 12.7% of sexual minority people were uninsured, but disability identity was not assessed.[39] We add valuable information about health insurance rates for those with disabilities. Our results pinpoint a growing area for improvement in public health outreach, pressing local, state, and federal agencies to target health insurance messaging that would help the SGM disability communities. Moreover, future investigations should address the relationship between health insurance and experiencing health care barriers.

Strengths and Limitations

Our study has several strengths. First, to the best of our knowledge, our study is the first to investigate health care access among SGM people with disabilities. Second, our study participants had diverse sexual orientations and gender identities, allowing the breadth of health care experiences and any barriers experienced. Third, the study sample was geographically diverse, drawing participants from the entire country. Fourth, in addition to describing the prevalence of SGM people with disabilities in our cohort, we differentiated the kinds of disabilities that were present, allowing greater understanding of the types of disabilities most prevalent.

There are also some limitations to our findings. First, although we classified disabilities into 4 categories, the heterogeneity in each category may have masked the distinctness of certain conditions. For instance, we classified attention deficit disorder as an intellectual or developmental disability; some may consider it a mental disability depending on the functional outcomes associated with the condition. Second, the race/ethnicity of the sample was predominantly White only, and The PRIDE Study is not a nationally representative sample because of recruitment efforts that were made by convenience sampling. These reasons may limit the generalizability of the results. Third, there was a lack of precision in defining disability severity. For example, there is variation in how much one's disability interferes with their daily life. Future investigations could assess disability severity and its relation to health care access. Fourth, there were no data on whether those with disabilities received any disability financial benefits. This information could help examine issues with affordability, which was brought up as a barrier. Fifth, we did not assess whether participants with cognitive or developmental disabilities answered the survey questions or whether someone assisted them; ensuring a participant's comprehension of the survey questions is necessary to capture responses from all groups of individuals and uphold equity.

Conclusions

We found that SGM people with disabilities experienced significant barriers in accessing health care services compared with those without disabilities. SGM people with disabilities were younger, racially/ethnically more diverse, less likely to be employed, less likely to have a usual health care provider, and more likely to have trouble finding a provider. SGM people with disabilities had an increased odds of delaying care and being unable to obtain health care in the past 12 months, which was markedly different from those without disabilities. Our data suggest a relationship between disability status and experiencing health care barriers among SGM people. Discrimination, bias, stigma, mistreatment, costs, and physical limitations can all influence the decisions to delay care. Overall, public health initiatives should be tailored to improve cultural competency and address insurance coverage for the SGM disability population. AJPH

ABOUT THE AUTHORS

Shane Lamba, Juno Obedin-Maliver, Annesa Flentje, Micah E. Lubensky, Zubin Dastur, and Mitchell R. Lunn are with The PRIDE Study/PRIDEnet, Stanford University School of Medicine, Stanford, CA. Jonathan Mayo is with the Dunlevie Maternal-Fetal Medicine Center, Stanford University School of Medicine.

CORRESPONDENCE

Correspondence should be sent to Mitchell R. Lunn, MD, MAS, 3180 Porter Dr, Suite B214, Palo Alto, CA 94304 (e-mail: lunn@stanford.edu). Reprints can be ordered at http://www.ajph.org by clicking the "Reprints" link.

PUBLICATION INFORMATION

Full Citation: Lamba S, Obedin-Maliver J, Mayo J, et al. Self-reported barriers to care among sexual and gender minority people with disabilities: findings from The Pride Study, 2019–2020. *Am J Public Health*. 2023;113(9):1009–1018.

Acceptance Date: May 8, 2023.

DOI: https://doi.org/10.2105/AJPH.2023.307333

CONTRIBUTORS

S. Lamba and M.R. Lunn conceptualized and designed the study and drafted the article. J. Obedin-Maliver, A. Flentje, and M.R. Lunn obtained funding. J. Mayo conducted the analyses. M.E. Lubensky and Z. Dastur were responsible for study operation, including participant experience and participant questions. All authors provided significant input, review, and editing and read and approved the final version of the article.

ACKNOWLEDGMENTS

Research reported in this article was partially funded through the Patient-Centered Outcomes Research Institute (PCORI; award PPRN-1501-26848 to M. R. L.). J. Obedin-Maliver was partially supported by the National Institute of Diabetes and Digestive and Kidney Diseases (grant K12DK111028). A. Flentje was partially supported by the National Institute on Drug Abuse (grant K23DA039800).

Data from this article were orally presented at AcademyHealth's Annual Research Meeting on June 4, 2022 in Washington, DC.

The PRIDE Study is a community-engaged research project that serves and is made possible by lesbian, gay, bisexual, transgender, and queer community involvement at multiple points in the research process, including the dissemination of findings. We acknowledge the courage and dedication of The PRIDE Study participants for sharing their stories and the careful attention of PRIDEnet Participant Advisory Committee members for reviewing and improving every study application.

Note. The statements in this article are solely the responsibility of the authors and do not necessarily represent the views of PCORI, its board of governors, or its methodology committee.

CONFLICTS OF INTEREST

S. Lamba, J. Mayo, A. Flentje, M.E. Lubensky, and Z. Dastur have no conflicts of interest to declare. J. Obedin-Maliver has consulted for Sage Therapeutics (May 2017) in a 1-day advisory board, Ibis Reproductive Health (a not-for-profit research group; March 2017–May 2018, 2020–present), Folx, Inc. (2020–present), and Hims, Inc. (2019–present). M.R. Lunn has consulted for Folx, Inc. (2020–2021) and Hims, Inc. (2019–present).

HUMAN PARTICIPANT PROTECTION

This study was reviewed and approved by the institutional review boards of Stanford University and the University of California, San Francisco. The PRIDE Study's Research Advisory Committee and Participant Advisory Committee reviewed and approved this ancillary study.

REFERENCES

1. Centers for Disease Control and Prevention. Prevalence of disabilities and health care access by disability status and type among adults—United States, 2016. *MMWR Morb Mortal*

Wkly Rep. 2018;67(32):882–887. https://doi.org/10.15585/mmwr.mm6732a3

2. Centers for Disease Control and Prevention. Surveillance for health care access and health services use, adults aged 18–64 years—Behavioral Risk Factor Surveillance System, United States, 2014. *MMWR Surveill Summ.* 2017;66(7):1–42. https://doi.org/10.15585/mmwr.ss6607a1
3. Casey R. Disability and unmet health care needs in Canada: a longitudinal analysis. *Disabil Health J.* 2015;8(2):173–181. https://doi.org/10.1016/j.dhjo.2014.09.010
4. Reichard A, Stransky M, Phillips K, McClain M, Drum C. Prevalence and reasons for delaying and foregoing necessary care by the presence and type of disability among working-age adults. *Disabil Health J.* 2017;10(1):39–47. https://doi.org/10.1016/j.dhjo.2016.08.001
5. Mahmoudi E, Meade MA. Disparities in access to health care among adults with physical disabilities: analysis of a representative national sample for a ten-year period. *Disabil Health J.* 2015; 8(2):182–190. https://doi.org/10.1016/j.dhjo.2014.08.007
6. Miller NA, Kirk A, Kaiser MJ, Glos L. The relation between health insurance and health care disparities among adults with disabilities. *Am J Public Health.* 2014;104(3):e85–e93. https://doi.org/10.2105/AJPH.2013.301478
7. Macapagal K, Bhatia R, Greene GJ. Differences in healthcare access, use, and experiences within a community sample of racially diverse lesbian, gay, bisexual, transgender, and questioning emerging adults. *LGBT Health.* 2016;3(6):434–442. https://doi.org/10.1089/lgbt.2015.0124
8. Progovac AM, Cook BL, Mullin BO, et al. Identifying gender minority patients' health and health care needs in administrative claims data. *Health Aff (Millwood).* 2018;37(3):413–420. https://doi.org/10.1377/hlthaff.2017.1295
9. Wingo E, Ingraham N, Roberts SCM. Reproductive health care priorities and barriers to effective care for LGBTQ people assigned female at birth: a qualitative study. *Womens Health Issues.* 2018;28(4):350–357. https://doi.org/10.1016/j.whi.2018.03.002
10. Eckhert E, Lansinger O, Ritter V, et al. Breast cancer diagnosis, treatment, and outcomes of patients from sex and gender minority groups. *JAMA Oncol.* 2023;9(4):473–480. https://doi.org/10.1001/jamaoncol.2022.7146
11. Jennings L, Barcelos C, McWilliams C, Malecki K. Inequalities in lesbian, gay, bisexual, and transgender (LGBT) health and health care access and utilization in Wisconsin. *Prev Med Rep.* 2019; 14:100864. https://doi.org/10.1016/j.pmedr.2019.100864
12. James SE, Herman JL, Rankin S, Keisling M, Mottet L, Anafi M. The report of the 2015 US Transgender Survey. 2016. Available at: https://transequality.org/sites/default/files/docs/usts/USTS-Full-Report-Dec17.pdf. Accessed May 20, 2023.
13. Conover KJ, Israel T. Microaggressions and social support among sexual minorities with physical disabilities. *Rehabil Psychol.* 2019;64(2):167–178. https://doi.org/10.1037/rep0000250
14. Eliason MJ, Martinson M, Carabez RM. Disability among sexual minority women: descriptive data from an invisible population. *LGBT Health.* 2015;2(2):113–120. https://doi.org/10.1089/lgbt.2014.0091
15. US Department of Health and Human Services. LGBT–Healthy People 2030. Available at: https://health.gov/healthypeople/objectives-and-data/browse-objectives/lgbt. Accessed July 6, 2022.
16. US Department of Health and Human Services. Health care access and quality—Healthy People 2030. Available at: https://health.gov/healthypeople/objectives-and-data/browse-objectives/health-care-access-and-quality. Accessed July 6, 2022.
17. Lunn MR, Lubensky M, Hunt C, et al. A digital health research platform for community engagement, recruitment, and retention of sexual and gender minority adults in a national longitudinal cohort study—The PRIDE Study. *J Am Med Inform Assoc.* 2019;26(8–9):737–748. https://doi.org/10.1093/jamia/ocz082
18. Centers for Disease Control and Prevention. Disability and health overview. September 15, 2020. Available at: https://www.cdc.gov/ncbddd/disabilityandhealth/disability.html. Accessed August 4, 2022.
19. National Center for Health Statistics. 2019 National Health Interview Survey Questionnaire. April 5, 2021. Available at: https://ftp.cdc.gov/pub/Health_Statistics/NCHS/Survey_Questionnaires/NHIS/2019/EnglishQuest.pdf. Accessed July 14, 2022.
20. US Department of Agriculture. Rural–urban commuting area (RUCA) documentation. August 17, 2020. Available at: https://www.ers.usda.gov/data-products/rural-urban-commuting-area-codes/documentation. Accessed February 13, 2023.
21. LaVaccare S, Diamant AL, Friedman J, et al. Healthcare experiences of underrepresented lesbian and bisexual women: a focus group qualitative study. *Health Equity.* 2018;2(1):131–138. https://doi.org/10.1089/heq.2017.0041
22. Marney HL, Vawdrey DK, Warsame L, et al. Overcoming technical and cultural challenges to delivering equitable care for LGBTQ+ individuals in a rural, underserved area. *J Am Med Inform Assoc.* 2021;29(2):372–378. https://doi.org/10.1093/jamia/ocab227
23. Mayer KH, Bradford JB, Makadon HJ, Stall R, Goldhammer H, Landers S. Sexual and gender minority health: what we know and what needs to be done. *Am J Public Health.* 2008;98(6):989–995. https://doi.org/10.2105/AJPH.2007.127811
24. Streed CG, Hall JP, Boyd BA, Batza K, Kurth NK. Comparative health status and characteristics of respondents of the 2019–2020 National Survey on Health and Disability by sexual and gender minority status. *LGBT Health.* 2021;8(8):563–568. https://doi.org/10.1089/lgbt.2021.0075
25. Centers for Disease Control and Prevention. Disability impacts all of us infographic. March 8, 2019. Available at: https://www.cdc.gov/ncbddd/disabilityandhealth/infographic-disability-impacts-all.html. Accessed November 4, 2020.
26. Kauth MR, Barrera TL, Latini DM. Lesbian, gay, and transgender veterans' experiences in the Veterans Health Administration: positive signs and room for improvement. *Psychol Serv.* 2019;16(2):346–351. https://doi.org/10.1037/ser0000232
27. Fredriksen-Goldsen KI, Kim HJ, Barkan SE. Disability among lesbian, gay, and bisexual adults: disparities in prevalence and risk. *Am J Public Health.* 2012;102(1):e16–e21. https://doi.org/10.2105/AJPH.2011.300379
28. Kaye HS. Disability-related disparities in access to health care before (2008–2010) and after (2015–2017) the Affordable Care Act. *Am J Public Health.* 2019;109(7):1015–1021. https://doi.org/10.2105/AJPH.2019.305056
29. Henning-Smith C, McAlpine D, Shippee T, Priebe M. Delayed and unmet need for medical care among publicly insured adults with disabilities. *Med Care.* 2013;51(11):1015–1019. https://doi.org/10.1097/MLR.0b013e3182a95d65
30. Kennedy J, Wood EG, Frieden L. Disparities in insurance coverage, health services use, and access following implementation of the Affordable Care Act: a comparison of disabled and nondisabled working-age adults. *Inquiry.* 2017;54:46958017734031. https://doi.org/10.1177/0046958017734031
31. Jones E, Pike J, Marshall T, Ye X. Quantifying the relationship between increased disability and health care resource utilization, quality of life, work productivity, health care costs in patients with multiple sclerosis in the US. *BMC Health Serv Res.* 2016;16:294. https://doi.org/10.1186/s12913-016-1532-1
32. Hall JP, Shartzer A, Kurth NK, Thomas KC. Medicaid expansion as an employment incentive program for people with disabilities. *Am J Public Health.* 2018;108(9):1235–1237. https://doi.org/10.2105/AJPH.2018.304536
33. Hall JP, Kurth NK, Gimm G, Smith S. Perspectives of adults with disabilities on access to health care after the ACA: qualitative findings. *Disabil Health J.* 2019;12(3):350–358. https://doi.org/10.1016/j.dhjo.2019.01.014
34. Waad A. Caring for our community: telehealth interventions as a promising practice for addressing population health disparities of LGBTQ+ communities in health care settings. *Dela J Public Health.* 2019;5(3):12–15.
35. Chen X, Orom H, Hay JL, et al. Differences in rural and urban health information access and use. *J Rural Health.* 2019;35(3):405–417. https://doi.org/10.1111/jrh.12335
36. Moscoso-Porras MG, Alvarado GF. Association between perceived discrimination and healthcare-seeking behavior in people with a disability. *Disabil Health J.* 2018;11(1):93–98. https://doi.org/10.1016/j.dhjo.2017.04.002
37. Ayhan CHB, Bilgin H, Uluman OT, Sukut O, Yilmaz S, Buzlu S. A systematic review of the discrimination against sexual and gender minority in health care settings. *Int J Health Serv.* 2020;50(1):44–61. https://doi.org/10.1177/0020731419885093
38. O'Shea A, Latham JR, McNair R, et al. Experiences of LGBTIQA+ people with disability in healthcare and community services: towards embracing multiple identities. *Int J Environ Res Public Health.* 2020;17(21):8080. https://doi.org/10.3390/ijerph17218080
39. Bosworth A, Turrini G, Pyda S, et al. Health insurance coverage and access to care for LGBTQ+ individuals: current trends and key challenges. June 2021. Available at: https://aspe.hhs.gov/sites/default/files/2021-07/lgbt-health-ib.pdf. Accessed January 24, 2022.

Benefits of Frequent HIV Testing in the THRIVE Demonstration Project: United States, 2015–2020

Anne A. Kimball, MD, MPH, Weiming Zhu, MD, PhD, Lei Yu, PhD, Mary R. Tanner, MD, Kashif Iqbal, MPH, Kenneth L. Dominguez, MD, MPH, Aparna Shankar, MPH, Kate Drezner, MPH, Karen Musgrove, PhD, MEd, Eric Mayes, William T. Robinson, PhD, Christina Schumacher, PhD, Kevin P. Delaney, PhD, Karen W. Hoover, MD, MPH, and the THRIVE Project Team

Objectives. To describe HIV testing among clients in the Targeted Highly Effective Interventions to Reverse the HIV Epidemic (THRIVE) demonstration project and evaluate testing frequency.

Methods. We identified factors associated with an average testing frequency of 180 days or less compared with more than 180 days using adjusted Poisson regression models. We performed the Kaplan–Meier survival analysis to compare time to diagnosis by testing frequency.

Results. Among 5710 clients with 2 or more tests and no preexposure prophylaxis (PrEP) prescription, 42.4% were tested frequently. Black/African American clients were 21% less likely and Hispanic/Latino clients were 18% less likely to be tested frequently than were White clients. Among 71 Black/African American and Hispanic/Latino cisgender men who have sex with men and transgender women with HIV diagnoses, those with frequent testing had a median time to diagnosis of 137 days, with a diagnostic testing yield of 1.5% compared with those tested less frequently, with 559 days and 0.8% yield.

Conclusions. HIV testing at least every 6 months resulted in earlier HIV diagnosis and was efficient. Persons in communities with high rates of HIV who are not on PrEP can benefit from frequent testing, and collaborative community approaches may help reduce disparities. (*Am J Public Health*. 2023;113(9): 1019–1027. https://doi.org/10.2105/AJPH.2023.307341)

AJPH September 2023, Vol 113, No. 9

In 2019, there were more than 36 000 persons diagnosed with HIV infection in the United States. About 70% of these diagnoses were among gay, bisexual, and other men who have sex with men (MSM) and transgender women (TGW).[1] Black/African American and Hispanic/Latino persons were disproportionately affected. An estimated 13% of US persons with HIV infection were undiagnosed in 2019.[2] One of the 4 pillars of the Ending the HIV Epidemic in the US initiative, launched by the US Department of Health and Human Services in 2019, is to diagnose all persons with HIV as early as possible.[3]

HIV testing is a key intervention throughout both the HIV prevention continuum and the HIV care continuum. It allows persons with HIV to be diagnosed, initiate antiretroviral treatment, and become virally suppressed, which have the individual health benefit of preserving immune function and the public health benefit of reduced HIV transmission.[4,5] HIV testing also identifies persons who do not have HIV but might benefit from preexposure prophylaxis (PrEP) to prevent HIV acquisition.[6]

Since 2006, the Centers for Disease Control and Prevention (CDC) has recommended HIV testing at least once for all persons aged 13 to 64 years and at least annually for persons whose behaviors, circumstances, or sexual networks may be associated with increased likelihood of HIV acquisition; these persons include sexually active MSM and TGW, sex partners of persons with HIV infection, persons who exchange sex for money or drugs, and persons who inject drugs and their sex partners.[7] The CDC recommends that providers consider more frequent testing, every 3 to 6 months, for sexually active MSM.[4] Additionally, the CDC recommends HIV testing every 2 to 3 months for persons using long-acting injectable or oral PrEP.[6] Persons who might benefit from frequent HIV testing may not seek or receive it because of lack of awareness of HIV risk and structural and social barriers, including stigma, fear, and lack of access.[8]

We describe HIV testing of clients in the Targeted Highly Effective Interventions to Reverse the HIV Epidemic (THRIVE) demonstration project from 2015 to 2020 in the United States. We identified factors associated with receipt of frequent HIV testing and calculated the incidence of HIV infection, time to diagnosis, and diagnostic testing yield per test to evaluate the effectiveness and efficiency of frequent testing in communities with high rates of HIV diagnoses.

METHODS

In the THRIVE demonstration project, the CDC funded 7 US health departments to develop and lead community collaboratives to provide comprehensive, culturally sensitive HIV prevention and care services for cisgender MSM and TGW in communities with high numbers of Black/African American or Hispanic/Latino MSM with HIV infection.[1,9,10] The 7 THRIVE recipients were health departments in Birmingham, Alabama; Baltimore, Maryland; New Orleans, Louisiana; New York, New York; Philadelphia, Pennsylvania; Hampton Roads, Virginia; and the District of Columbia. Recipients collected longitudinal client-level data, including HIV testing and PrEP service provision, and reported de-identified data to the CDC for evaluation of the effectiveness of THRIVE. We considered anyone who received a THRIVE-funded service, including HIV and sexual health services and essential support services, a THRIVE client.

Inclusion Criteria

To describe HIV testing patterns in THRIVE, we included all clients who were aged 18 years or older, received an HIV test, and had a negative result on their first HIV test conducted in THRIVE. To estimate the frequency of testing, HIV incidence rates, and time to diagnosis, we included only clients who received 2 or more tests and excluded those who were prescribed PrEP in THRIVE, because persons using PrEP have a decreased risk of acquiring HIV and, per the CDC, should be tested for HIV every 2 to 3 months, depending on the type of PrEP.[6]

Definitions

We assessed the race/ethnicity, gender identity, and sexual behaviors of clients because these characteristics are associated with increased rates of HIV diagnoses, understanding that race/ethnicity may serve as a proxy for underlying social, environmental, and structural factors, including systemic racism.[1,11] We categorized age groups by clients' age at enrollment as 18 to 24, 25 to 34, 35 to 44, 45 to 54, and 55 or older years. We determined racial/ethnic group by client self-reported race and ethnicity and categorized it as Hispanic/Latino (including persons of any race), Black/African American, White, other race (including persons who identified as American Indian/Alaska Native, Asian, Native Hawaiian/other Pacific Islander, multiracial, or another race), and unknown. We determined clients' gender identity and sexual behavior group by client self-report and categorized it as cisgender MSM, TGW, transgender men, cisgender heterosexual men, cisgender women, and other (including clients who could not be assigned to 1 of the categories because of missing data). We categorized cisgender men as MSM or heterosexual based on whether they reported having sex with men. We did not stratify other gender identity groups by sexual behavior because of the small numbers of persons in these groups.

Estimating Testing Frequency

We included all types of HIV tests and identified unique testing events with a minimum gap of 20 days between 2 tests, accounting for the HIV infection window period.[12] We categorized clients with 2 tests performed less than 20 days apart as having 1 HIV test. We defined frequent testing as an average interval of 180 days or less between tests and less frequent testing as an interval of more than 180 days.

Statistical Analyses

We calculated the percentage increase in the number of HIV antigen/antibody tests performed, including lab-based and point-of-care tests. We described characteristics of THRIVE clients with an initial negative HIV test result stratified by receipt of only 1 HIV test and 2 or more tests. We also described characteristics of clients with 2 or more HIV tests who were not prescribed PrEP, stratified by frequency of HIV testing. We estimated adjusted risk ratios (ARRs) and 95% confidence intervals (CIs) using Poisson regression models for the association between client characteristics and frequency of testing. We adjusted for THRIVE site, age group, race/ethnicity group, and gender identity and sexual behavior group. We included THRIVE site as a covariate because of differences in the size and capacity of each program, as well as different social, cultural, and structural contexts in the communities served at each site.

To estimate the incidence rate of HIV diagnosis, we identified THRIVE clients who were not prescribed PrEP who had an initial negative HIV test result followed by a positive test result with at least 20 days between tests. We described the number of clients with HIV diagnoses, cumulative follow-up time for each person with 2 or more tests, incidence rate per 100 person-years of follow-up time, median number of tests per client, median interval between tests, and diagnostic testing yield per test stratified by race/ethnicity group and gender identity and sexual behavior group. We calculated the cumulative follow-up time for clients diagnosed with HIV with the time interval between the first date of testing and the first positive test date. For clients with no positive tests, we calculated the cumulative follow-up time as the gap between the first and last date of testing plus 90 days of potential continued enrollment, as clients would not be expected to receive another HIV test for at least 3 months.

We calculated the median number of tests for clients who had only negative tests using all testing data collected and for clients diagnosed with HIV infection using all testing data collected up until the positive test. We calculated the incidence rate per 100 person-years by dividing the number of new diagnoses by the cumulative follow-up time per person-years. We calculated the testing yield per HIV test by dividing the number of new diagnoses by the number of tests performed among clients.

For Black/African American and Hispanic/Latino cisgender MSM and TGW, the groups with the highest incidence of HIV in THRIVE, we performed the Kaplan–Meier survival analysis and used log-rank testing to compare the time to diagnosis between clients who received frequent testing and those who received less frequent testing. We assessed time to diagnosis as the time interval between the first negative test and the first positive test among persons diagnosed with HIV infection. We determined the median time to diagnosis among Black/African American and Hispanic/Latino cisgender MSM and TGW diagnosed with HIV infection and compared persons who received frequent testing with those who received less frequent testing. We performed all analyses using SAS version 9.4 (SAS Institute, Cary, NC) and prepared figures using R version 4.1.1 (RStudio, Boston, MA).

RESULTS

Overall, THRIVE provided HIV testing for 29 687 clients with an initial negative HIV test (Table 1). The number of lab-based antigen/antibody HIV tests performed in THRIVE increased 253%, from 2256 in 2016 to 7953 in 2019, and the number of point-of-care antigen/antibody tests increased 449%, from 1171 to 6427. Most clients (71.7%) received only 1 HIV test, and this did not vary by age or race/ethnicity. Almost half of cisgender MSM (4653; 44.2%) and more than half of TGW (429; 51.9%) received 2 or more tests.

Among 5710 clients who received 2 or more HIV tests and were not prescribed PrEP (Figure A, available as a supplement to the online version of this article at http://www.ajph.org), 42.4% received frequent HIV testing (Table 2). Clients aged 18 to 24 years were more likely to receive frequent testing than were those aged 35 to 44 years, with an ARR of 1.15 (95% CI = 1.01, 1.31), after adjusting for THRIVE site, race/ethnicity group, and gender identity and sexual behavior group. Compared with White clients, Black/African American clients were 21% less likely to receive frequent testing (ARR = 0.79; 95% CI = 0.70, 0.90) and Hispanic/Latino clients were 18% less likely (ARR = 0.82; 95% CI = 0.70, 0.96). Compared with cisgender heterosexual men, MSM were 25% more likely to receive frequent testing (ARR = 1.25; 95% CI = 1.11, 1.41), TGW were 24% more likely (ARR = 1.24; 95% CI = 0.99, 1.54), and cisgender women were 15% more likely (ARR = 1.15; 95% CI = 1.01, 1.31).

Among all 5710 clients, 92 were diagnosed with HIV infection while enrolled in THRIVE during 8432.2 observed person-years, with an incidence rate of 1.1 per 100 person-years (Table 3). Among 92 clients diagnosed with HIV infection, 72 were cisgender MSM, 6 were TGW, 6 were cisgender women, and 8 were cisgender heterosexual men (Table 3; Table A, available as a supplement to the online version of this article at http://www.ajph.org). The highest incidence rates were among cisgender MSM (2.0 per 100 person-years) and TGW (1.7 per 100 person-years). By known race/ethnicity group, the highest incidence rates were observed among Black/African American TGW (3.7 per 100 person-years), Black/African American MSM (3.1 per 100 person-years), and Hispanic/Latino MSM (1.9 per 100 person-years). The diagnostic testing yield per HIV test was highest among Black/African American TGW (1.6%), Black/African American MSM (1.4%), and Hispanic/Latino MSM (0.8%).

Among 1819 Black/African American and Hispanic/Latino cisgender MSM and TGW, 71 were diagnosed with HIV infection during an observed

AJPH September 2023, Vol 113, No. 9

TABLE 1— Characteristics of Clients Enrolled in THRIVE by the Number of HIV Tests: United States, 2015–2020

	Clients, No. (%)		
	Total	1 HIV Test[a]	≥2 HIV Tests[b]
Total	29 687	21 289	8 398
Age group, y			
18–24	8 223	6 069 (28.5)	2 154 (25.6)
25–34	11 086	7 458 (35.0)	3 628 (43.2)
35–44	5 081	3 590 (16.9)	1 491 (17.8)
45–54	2 868	2 192 (10.3)	676 (8.0)
≥55	2 398	1 959 (9.2)	439 (5.2)
Unknown/missing	31	21 (0.1)	10 (0.1)
Race/ethnicity			
White	4 341	3 259 (15.3)	1 082 (12.9)
Black/African American	18 341	13 537 (63.6)	4 804 (57.2)
Hispanic/Latino[c]	4 603	2 916 (13.7)	1 687 (20.1)
Other[d]	1 709	1 070 (5.0)	639 (7.6)
Unknown	693	507 (2.4)	186 (2.2)
Gender identity/sexual behavior			
Cisgender MSM	10 526	5 873 (27.6)	4 653 (55.4)
TGW	827	398 (1.9)	429 (5.1)
TGM	287	169 (0.8)	118 (1.4)
Cisgender women	8 729	7 285 (34.2)	1 444 (17.2)
Cisgender heterosexual men	9 099	7 393 (34.7)	1 706 (20.3)
Other[e]	219	171 (0.8)	48 (0.6)
Prescribed PrEP			
Yes	3 887	1 199 (5.6)	2 688 (32.0)
No	25 800	20 090 (94.4)	5 710 (68.0)

Note. MSM = gay, bisexual, and other men who have sex with men; PrEP = preexposure prophylaxis; TGM = transgender men; TGW = transgender women; THRIVE = Targeted Highly Effective Interventions to Reverse the HIV Epidemic demonstration project.

[a]Includes clients with only 1 HIV test with a negative result. Only tests > 20 d apart were considered to be independent testing events.
[b]Includes clients with ≥ 2 HIV tests among those with an initial negative HIV test and > 20 d between tests.
[c]Hispanic/Latino clients can be of any race.
[d]Other includes clients who self-identified as American Indian/Alaska Native, Asian, Native Hawaiian/other Pacific Islander, and other.
[e]Includes clients with missing gender identity or sexual behavior variables.

2717.4 person-years, with an incidence rate of 2.6 per 100 person-years and a testing yield of 1.2% per test. Among these clients, 71.8% received frequent testing. The testing yield per test among clients with frequent testing was 1.5% compared with a testing yield of 0.8% among those with less frequent testing. Clients with frequent testing had a shorter time to diagnosis (or end of follow-up period) than did those who received less frequent testing ($P < .001$). Clients diagnosed with HIV infection who received frequent testing had a shorter median time to diagnosis (137 days; IQR = 83–503) than did those who received less frequent testing (559 days; IQR = 311–709; Figure 1).

DISCUSSION

THRIVE successfully implemented sensitive antigen/antibody HIV testing for the priority populations of cisgender MSM and TGW. Black/African American and Hispanic/Latino MSM and TGW had the highest HIV incidence rates in THRIVE, mirroring the epidemiology of HIV in the United States.[1] Among this group of THRIVE clients with high incidence rates, we found that clients with frequent testing had shorter time to diagnosis than did those who tested less frequently. Frequent testing was also efficient, with a high diagnostic testing yield per test among tests performed in

TABLE 2— Characteristics Associated With Frequent Testing Among THRIVE Clients With ≥ 2 HIV Tests and Not Prescribed PrEP: United States, 2015–2020

	Clients, No. (%)			
	Total[a]	Testing Frequency of > 180 d[b]	Testing Frequency of ≤ 180 d[c]	ARR (95% CI)[d]
Total	5 710	3 289 (57.6)	2 421 (42.4)	
Age group at enrollment, y				
18–24	1 747	982 (56.2)	765 (43.8)	1.15 (1.01, 1.31)
25–34	2 287	1 288 (56.3)	999 (43.7)	1.10 (0.97, 1.24)
35–44	907	543 (59.9)	364 (40.1)	1 (Ref)
45–54	433	261 (60.3)	172 (39.7)	1.04 (0.86, 1.24)
≥ 55	334	214 (64.1)	120 (35.9)	0.97 (0.79, 1.19)
Unknown/missing	2	1 (50.0)	1 (50.0)	1.27 (0.18, 9.05)
Race/ethnicity				
White	730	286 (39.2)	444 (60.8)	1 (Ref)
Black/African American	3 633	2 293 (63.1)	1 340 (36.9)	0.79 (0.70, 0.90)
Hispanic/Latino[e]	918	486 (52.9)	432 (47.1)	0.82 (0.70, 0.96)
Other[f]	329	170 (51.7)	159 (48.3)	0.85 (0.70, 1.04)
Unknown	100	54 (54.0)	46 (46.0)	0.78 (0.57, 1.07)
Gender identity/sexual behavior				
Cisgender MSM	2 465	1 190 (48.3)	1 275 (51.7)	1.25 (1.11, 1.41)
TGW	225	116 (51.6)	109 (48.4)	1.24 (0.99, 1.54)
TGM	93	55 (59.1)	38 (40.9)	1.00 (0.71, 1.41)
Cisgender women	1 328	825 (62.1)	503 (37.9)	1.15 (1.01, 1.31)
Cisgender heterosexual men	1 566	1 085 (69.3)	481 (30.7)	1 (Ref)
Other[g]	33	18 (54.5)	15 (45.5)	1.07 (0.64, 1.80)

Note. ARR = adjusted risk ratio; CI = confidence interval; MSM = gay, bisexual, and other men who have sex with men; PrEP = preexposure prophylaxis; TGM = transgender men; TGW = transgender women; THRIVE = Targeted Highly Effective Interventions to Reverse the HIV Epidemic demonstration project.

[a]Includes clients with ≥ 2 HIV tests > 20 d apart among those with an initial negative HIV test result and not prescribed PrEP in THRIVE.
[b]Less frequent testing was defined as an average interval of > 180 d between tests.
[c]Frequent testing was defined as an average interval of ≤ 180 d between tests.
[d]Adjusted for THRIVE site, age group, racial/ethnic group, and gender identity/sexual behavior group.
[e]Hispanic/Latino clients can be of any race.
[f]Other includes clients who self-identified as American Indian/Alaska Native, Asian, Native Hawaiian/other Pacific Islander, and other.
[g]Includes clients with missing gender identity/sexual behavior variables.

this group. These findings can inform HIV testing recommendations for persons not using PrEP and can serve as inputs in modeling studies of HIV transmission and cost-effectiveness.

Despite implementation of culturally sensitive programs, Black/African American and Hispanic/Latino THRIVE clients were less likely to receive frequent testing than were White clients, underscoring ongoing disparities in HIV prevention that were not eliminated during the project period. Persons in racial and ethnic minority groups and sexual and gender minority groups who are disproportionately affected by HIV, and who may benefit most from frequent HIV testing, often encounter social and structural barriers that adversely affect their health.[13] These social and structural factors, including systemic racism, poverty, stigma, and discrimination, prevent equity in receipt of HIV prevention services.[8,14] Collaborative, culturally sensitive, community-tailored programs like THRIVE can increase the use of HIV testing and PrEP and can help to reduce disparities,[15] but additional large-scale and long-term interventions may be needed to overcome the long-standing, deeply rooted barriers that drive disparities.

THRIVE successfully engaged a large number of MSM and TGW in HIV testing, the first step in receipt of HIV prevention and care services.

AJPH September 2023, Vol 113, No. 9

TABLE 3— Clients Diagnosed With HIV Infection, Incidence Rate, and Testing Yield in THRIVE: United States, 2015–2020

Gender Identity, Sexual Behavior, and Race/Ethnicity Group	No. Clients With ≥2 HIV Tests[a]	No. Clients With New HIV Diagnoses	Follow-Up Time, Person-Years	Incidence Rate per 100 Person-Years	No. HIV Tests	Median No. of Tests (IQR)	Median No. of Days Between Tests (IQR)	Diagnostic Testing Yield per Test,[b] %
Total	5710	92	8432.2	1.1	17401	2 (2–3)	150 (91–288)	0.53
Cisgender MSM	2465	72	3544.5	2.0	8357	3 (2–4)	119 (80–233)	0.86
White	562	2	758.6	0.3	2038	3 (2–4)	98 (77–181)	0.10
Black/African American	1069	49	1596.3	3.1	3532	2 (2–4)	137 (83–257)	1.39
Hispanic/Latino[c]	568	16	829.0	1.9	1912	2 (2–4)	124 (82–246)	0.84
Other race[d]	218	2	308.7	0.6	752	3 (2–4)	112 (75–222)	0.27
Unknown	48	3	52.0	5.8	123	2 (2–3)	175 (98–310)	2.44
TGW	225	6	358.3	1.7	828	3 (2–4)	138 (88–231)	0.72
White	15	0	18.5	0.0	49	2 (2–5)	113 (70–205)	0.00
Black/African American	87	5	134.5	3.7	304	3 (2–4)	147 (96–227)	1.64
Hispanic/Latino[c]	95	1	157.6	0.6	362	3 (2–5)	134 (87–235)	0.28
Other[d]	15	0	26.9	0.0	51	3 (2–4)	183 (113–340)	0.00
Unknown	13	0	20.8	0.0	62	4 (2–5)	92 (70–142)	0.00
TGM	93	0	145.5	0.0	298	3 (2–4)	156 (98–298)	0.00
White	6	0	6.6	0.0	15	2 (2–3)	154 (119–342)	0.00
Black/African American	46	0	79.0	0.0	149	3 (2–4)	188 (119–308)	0.00
Hispanic/Latino[c]	24	0	37.8	0.0	89	2.5 (2–5)	105 (76–247)	0.00
Other[d]	7	0	9.3	0.0	14	2 (2–2)	378 (168–595)	0.00
Unknown	10	0	12.8	0.0	31	3 (2–4)	140 (98–252)	0.00
Cisgender women	1328	6	1882.5	0.3	3577	2 (2–3)	183 (104–341)	0.17
White	74	1	78.0	1.3	168	2 (2–2)	178 (103–304)	0.60
Black/African American	1100	5	1604.2	0.3	3026	2 (2–3)	182 (104–337)	0.17
Hispanic/Latino[c]	102	0	138.0	0.0	260	2 (2–3)	206 (102–364)	0.00
Other[d]	37	0	45.7	0.0	85	2 (2–2)	196 (141–404)	0.00
Unknown	15	0	16.6	0.0	38	2 (2–3)	182 (88–241)	0.00
Cisgender heterosexual men	1566	8	2453.4	0.3	4232	2 (2–3)	210 (113–370)	0.19
White	64	0	70.2	0.0	147	2 (2–2)	197 (96–312)	0.00
Black/African American	1320	7	2109.1	0.3	3559	2 (2–3)	217 (119–379)	0.20
Hispanic/Latino[c]	121	1	189.1	0.5	357	2 (2–3)	165 (91–329)	0.28
Other[d]	52	0	72.2	0.0	147	2 (2–3)	139 (88–308)	0.00
Unknown	9	0	12.8	0.0	22	2 (2–3)	206 (127–307)	0.00

Continued

TABLE 3— Continued

Gender Identity, Sexual Behavior, and Race/Ethnicity Group	No. Clients With ≥2 HIV Tests[a]	No. Clients With New HIV Diagnoses	Follow-Up Time, Person-Years	Incidence Rate per 100 Person-Years	No. HIV Tests	Median No. of Tests (IQR)	Median No. of Days Between Tests (IQR)	Diagnostic Testing Yield per Test,[b] %
Black/African American and Hispanic/Latino cisgender MSM and TGW	1 819	71	2 717.4	2.6	6 110	3 (2–4)	133 (83, 251)	1.20
Frequent testing[e]	860	51	1 025.3	5.0	3 496	3 (2–5)	98 (66, 143)	1.50
Less frequent testing[f]	959	20	1 692.1	1.2	2 614	2 (2–3)	278 (181, 432)	0.80

Note. IQR = interquartile range; MSM = gay, bisexual, and other men who have sex with men; TGM = transgender men; TGW = transgender women; THRIVE = Targeted Highly Effective Interventions to Reverse the HIV Epidemic demonstration project.

[a]Includes clients with ≥ 2 HIV tests > 20 d apart among those with an initial negative HIV test result and not prescribed preexposure prophylaxis in THRIVE.
[b]Testing yield per HIV test was calculated by dividing the number of new diagnoses by the number of tests among clients.
[c]Hispanic/Latino clients can be of any race.
[d]Other includes clients who self-identified as American Indian/Alaska Native, Asian, Native Hawaiian/other Pacific Islander, and other.
[e]Frequent testing was defined as an average interval of ≤ 180 days between tests.
[f]Less frequent testing was defined as an average interval of > 180 days between tests.

Frequent testing resulted in earlier diagnosis of HIV infection, which has both individual and public health benefits. Early initiation of antiretroviral therapy supports viral suppression, leading to reduced HIV-related morbidity and mortality and prevention of community transmission.[4,5] A negative HIV test is an opportunity to discuss HIV prevention options and, when appropriate, to start PrEP.[6] Although many MSM and TGW were tested frequently in THRIVE, large proportions received only 1 HIV test or were tested less frequently.

Interventions are needed to increase HIV testing coverage and frequency of testing of persons in communities with a high prevalence of HIV or with behaviors associated with HIV acquisition. Among MSM and TGW, about 20% self-reported that they had not received an HIV test in the previous 12 months.[16] A nationally representative study of visits to ambulatory health care providers found that HIV testing must increase at least threefold among US men to provide universal testing coverage.[17] Increasing routine HIV testing coverage and increasing the frequency of testing among persons with risk factors will require interventions in both clinical and public health settings. Innovative strategies include self-test kit distribution and clinical decision support tools that are programmed in electronic health record systems to generate automated test orders.[13,18,19] Community-based programs that are tailored for the local context may also help to increase frequent HIV testing among persons who may benefit.

Limitations

Although this analysis has many strengths, including an analysis of longitudinal data from a large cohort of

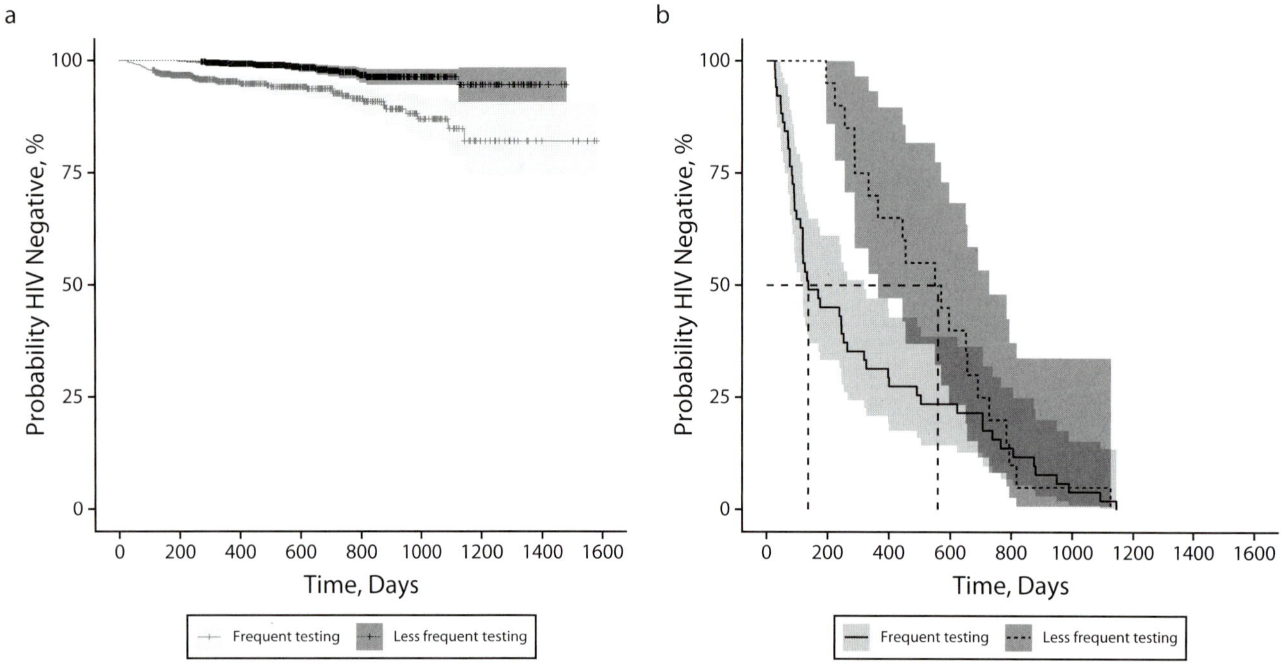

FIGURE 1— Time to Diagnosis of HIV Infection or End of Follow-Up and Frequency of Testing Among Black/African American and Hispanic/Latino Cisgender Gay, Bisexual, and Other Men Who Have Sex With Men (MSM) and Transgender Women (TGW) Who (a) Had ≥ 2 HIV Tests > 20 Days Apart, Had an Initial Negative HIV Test Result, and Were Not Prescribed Preexposure Prophylaxis; and (b) Were Diagnosed With HIV Infection: THRIVE, United States, 2015–2020

Note. THRIVE = Targeted Highly Effective Interventions to Reverse the HIV Epidemic demonstration project. The sample size in part a was n = 1819; we used a log-rank test to compare the time to diagnosis between those with frequent and those with less frequent testing ($P < .001$). The sample size in part b was n = 71. Dashed lines represent median time to diagnosis. The median time to diagnosis among persons with frequent testing was 137 days (interquartile range [IQR] = 83–503) and among persons with less frequent testing was 559 days (IQR = 311–709).

Black/African American and Hispanic/Latino MSM and TGW, it has at least 4 limitations. First, we were unable to evaluate clients' behaviors that might be associated with acquisition of HIV, such as frequency of sexual and injection drug use behaviors, because these data were not collected in THRIVE. If a client disclosed behaviors to their provider, they might have been tested more frequently. We were also unable to assess clients' intent or motivation for testing and whether the clients' health care providers recommended HIV testing. Given the high rates of persons diagnosed with HIV infection in the priority populations served by THRIVE, we assumed that most clients were at substantial risk of acquiring HIV and would probably have benefited from frequent testing.

Second, in this analysis, we could not assess whether a client received an HIV test or an HIV diagnosis outside the THRIVE collaborative, as data were collected only on the services provided by members of the collaborative, so we might have underestimated the proportion of clients who were frequently tested or diagnosed with HIV. Third, if a client's gender identity and sexual behavior group was misclassified, we might have underestimated the number of Black/African American and Hispanic/Latino cisgender MSM and TGW who were tested. If clients experienced differential levels of stigma, certain gender identities and sexual behaviors might have been underreported. Fourth, HIV testing patterns observed in THRIVE may not be generalizable to other populations, communities, or geographic locations.

Public Health Implications

HIV testing is the first step to receipt of HIV prevention and care services. Frequent HIV testing, at least every 6 months, identified HIV infections earlier, with shorter time to diagnosis, and was efficient, with high testing yield for persons in the priority populations who are disproportionately affected by HIV. Although interventions were implemented in THRIVE jurisdictions to increase community collaboration and to provide culturally sensitive and community-tailored HIV prevention services, we observed disparities in the frequency of HIV testing. Additional long-term, multifaceted programs may be needed to increase HIV testing among persons in priority populations and to overcome the social and structural barriers that drive disparities in HIV incidence. AJPH

ABOUT THE AUTHORS

Anne A. Kimball, Weiming Zhu, Mary R. Tanner, Kashif Iqbal, Kenneth L. Dominguez, Kevin P. Delaney, and Karen W. Hoover are with the Division of HIV Prevention, Centers for Disease Control and Prevention, Atlanta, GA. Lei Yu is with the DLH Corporation, Atlanta. Aparna Shankar is with the New York City Department of Health and Mental Hygiene, New York, NY. Kate Drezner is with the District of Columbia Department of Health, Washington, DC. Karen Musgrove is with Birmingham AIDS Outreach, Birmingham, AL. Eric Mayes is with the Virginia Department of Health, Richmond. William T. Robinson is with the Louisiana Office of Public Health and Louisiana State University Health Sciences Center, New Orleans. Christina Schumacher is with the Center for Child and Community Health Research, Johns Hopkins School of Medicine, Baltimore, MD.

CORRESPONDENCE

Correspondence should be sent to Karen W. Hoover, Centers for Disease Control and Prevention, 1600 Clifton Rd NE, Atlanta, GA 30329 (e-mail: khoover@cdc.gov). Reprints can be ordered at http://www.ajph.org by clicking the "Reprints" link.

PUBLICATION INFORMATION

Full Citation: Kimball AA, Zhu W, Yu L, et al. Benefits of frequent HIV testing in the THRIVE demonstration project: United States, 2015–2020. *Am J Public Health*. 2023;113(9):1019–1027.

Acceptance Date: May 16, 2023.

DOI: https://doi.org/10.2105/AJPH.2023.307341

CONTRIBUTORS

A. A. Kimball drafted and revised the article. A. A. Kimball and W. Zhu assisted with the analysis. A. A. Kimball, W. Zhu, K. P. Delaney, and K. W. Hoover conceptualized and designed the study. W. Zhu reviewed the analysis. W. Zhu, L. Yu, M. R. Tanner, K. Iqbal, K. L. Dominguez, A. Shankar, K. Drezner, K. Musgrove, E. Mayes, W. T. Robinson, C. Schumacher, K. P. Delaney, and K. W. Hoover critically reviewed the article for important intellectual content. L. Yu performed the analysis. M. R. Tanner, K. Iqbal, K. L. Dominguez, A. Shankar, K. Drezner, K. Musgrove, E. Mayes, W. T. Robinson, and C. Schumacher contributed to study design and data interpretation and assisted with data collection and with design and implementation of the demonstration project that generated the data. All authors approved publication of the final version of the article and agreed to be accountable for all aspects of the work.

ACKNOWLEDGMENTS

This work was supported by the Centers for Disease Control and Prevention (CDC) and the Minority HIV/AIDS Fund (cooperative agreement PS15-1509).

We would like to acknowledge contributors to this article from the Targeted Highly Effective Interventions to Reverse the HIV Epidemic (THRIVE) Project team: Benjamin Tsoi, Anthony Fox, Kenneth Pettigrew, Michael Kharfen, Jacquelyn Bickham, Anthony James, and Jacky Jennings.

Note. The findings and conclusions in this article are those of the authors and do not necessarily represent the official position of the CDC.

CONFLICTS OF INTEREST

The authors have no conflicts of interest to disclose.

HUMAN PARTICIPANT PROTECTION

The Centers for Disease Control and Prevention determined the THRIVE demonstration project to be nonresearch and exempt from institutional review board review.

REFERENCES

1. Centers for Disease Control and Prevention. Diagnoses of HIV infection in the United States and dependent areas 2019. Available at: https://www.cdc.gov/hiv/library/reports/hiv-surveillance/vol-32/index.html. Accessed March 10, 2022.
2. US Department of Health and Human Services. AHEAD: America's HIV epidemic analysis dashboard. Available at: https://ahead.hiv.gov. Accessed March 11, 2022.
3. Centers for Disease Control and Prevention. Ending the HIV epidemic in the US (EHE). Available at: https://www.cdc.gov/endhiv/index.html. Accessed March 10, 2022.
4. Centers for Disease Control and Prevention. Recommendations for HIV screening of gay, bisexual, and other men who have sex with men—United States, 2017. *MMWR Morb Mortal Wkly Rep*. 2017;66(31):830–832. https://doi.org/10.15585/mmwr.mm6631a3
5. Cohen MS, Chen YQ, McCauley M, et al. Antiretroviral therapy for the prevention of HIV-1 transmission. *N Engl J Med*. 2016;375(9):830–839. https://doi.org/10.1056/NEJMoa1600693
6. Centers for Disease Control and Prevention. *Preexposure Prophylaxis for the Prevention of HIV Infection in the United States—2021 Update: A Clinical Practice Guideline*. December 2021. Available at: https://www.cdc.gov/hiv/pdf/risk/prep/cdc-hiv-prep-guidelines-2021.pdf. Accessed March 10, 2022.
7. Centers for Disease Control and Prevention. Revised recommendations for HIV testing of adults, adolescents, and pregnant women in health-care settings. *MMWR Recomm Rep*. 2006;55(RR-14):1–17; quiz CE1-4. Available at: https://www.cdc.gov/mmwr/preview/mmwrhtml/rr5514a1.htm. Accessed June 22, 2023.
8. Kobrak P, Remien RH, Myers JE, et al. Motivations and barriers to routine HIV testing among men who have sex with men in New York City. *AIDS Behav*. 2022;26(11):3563–3575. https://doi.org/10.1007/s10461-022-03679-5
9. Centers for Disease Control and Prevention. THRIVE. Available at: https://www.cdc.gov/hiv/research/thrive/index.html. Accessed March 10, 2022.
10. Tanner MR, Iqbal K, Dominguez KL, Zhu W, Obi J, Hoover KW. Key factors for successful implementation of HIV prevention services by THRIVE community collaboratives. *Public Health Rep*. 2022;137(2):310–316. https://doi.org/10.1177/00333549211005793
11. Boyd RW, Lindo EG, Weeks LD, McLemore MR. On racism: a new standard for publishing on racial health inequities. July 2, 2020. Available at: https://www.healthaffairs.org/do/10.1377/forefront.20200630.939347/full. Accessed March 10, 2022.
12. Centers for Disease Control and Prevention. Understanding the HIV window period. 2022. Available at: https://www.cdc.gov/hiv/basics/hiv-testing/hiv-window-period.html. Accessed June 28, 2022.
13. Andrasik M, Broder G, Oseso L, Wallace S, Rentas F, Corey L. Stigma, implicit bias, and long-lasting prevention interventions to end the domestic HIV/AIDS epidemic. *Am J Public Health*. 2020;110(1):67–68. https://doi.org/10.2105/AJPH.2019.305454
14. Centers for Disease Control and Prevention. Estimated annual number of HIV infections—United States, 1981–2019. *MMWR Morb Mortal Wkly Rep*. 2021;70(22):801–806. https://doi.org/10.15585/mmwr.mm7022a1
15. Tanner MR, Zhu W, Iqbal K, et al. HIV Preexposure prophylaxis services for Black and Hispanic/Latino gay, bisexual, and other men who have sex with men and transgender women in THRIVE, 2015–2020. *J Acquir Immune Defic Syndr*. 2023;92(4):286–292. https://doi.org/10.1097/QAI.0000000000003138
16. Centers for Disease Control and Prevention. National HIV behavioral surveillance reports on men who have sex with men and transgender women. Available at: https://www.cdc.gov/hiv/statistics/systems/nhbs/index.html. Accessed June 28, 2022.
17. Hoover KW, Khalil GM, Cadwell BL, Rose CE, Peters PJ. Benchmarks for HIV testing: what is needed to achieve universal testing coverage at US ambulatory healthcare facilities. *J Acquir Immune Defic Syndr*. 2021;86(2):e48–e53. https://doi.org/10.1097/QAI.0000000000002553
18. Katz DA, Golden MR, Hughes JP, Farquhar C, Stekler JD. HIV self-testing increases HIV testing frequency in high-risk men who have sex with men: a randomized controlled trial. *J Acquir Immune Defic Syndr*. 2018;78(5):505–512. https://doi.org/10.1097/QAI.0000000000001709
19. Marcelin JR, Tan EM, Marcelin A, et al. Assessment and improvement of HIV screening rates in a Midwest primary care practice using an electronic clinical decision support system: a quality improvement study. *BMC Med Inform Decis Mak*. 2016;16:76. https://doi.org/10.1186/s12911-016-0320-5

Erratum In: "Beyond #StopAAPIHate: Expanding the Definition of Violence Against Asian Americans"

In: Fan CA. Beyond #StopAAPIHate: expanding the definition of violence against Asian Americans. *Am J Public Health*. 2022;112(4):604–606.

When originally published, the online version of the article listed the incorrect correspondence information. Correspondence should be sent to Carolyn A. Fan, BA, Department of Health Systems and Population Health, University of Washington School of Public Health, 1959 NE Pacific St, Magnuson Health Sciences Center, Seattle, WA, 98195 (e-mail: cfan5@uw.edu).

This change does not affect the article's conclusions. AJPH

https://doi.org/10.2105/AJPH.2022.306740e

GET DOWN
WITH YOUR BLOOD PRESSURE™

1

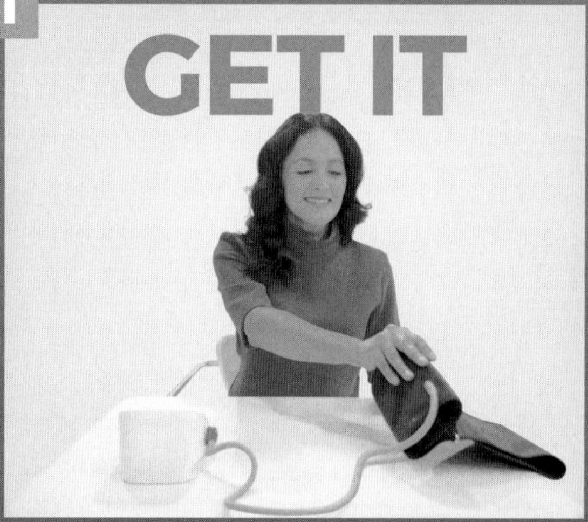

2

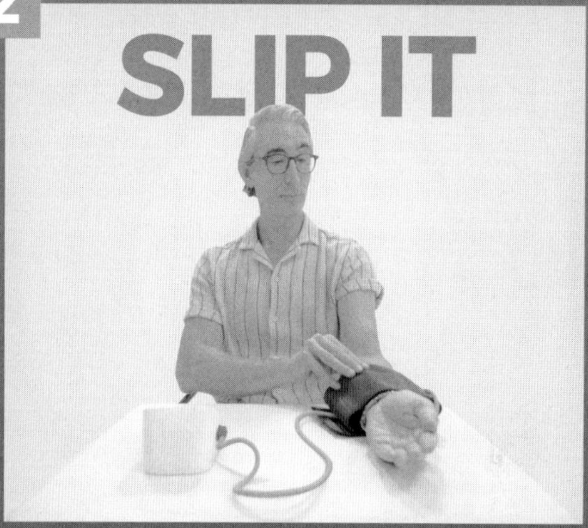

3

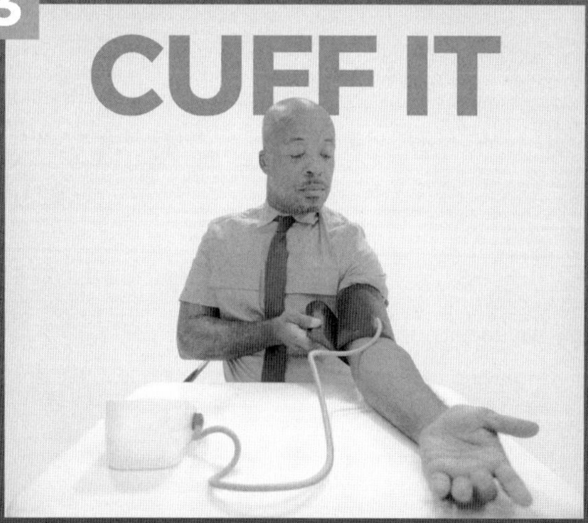

4

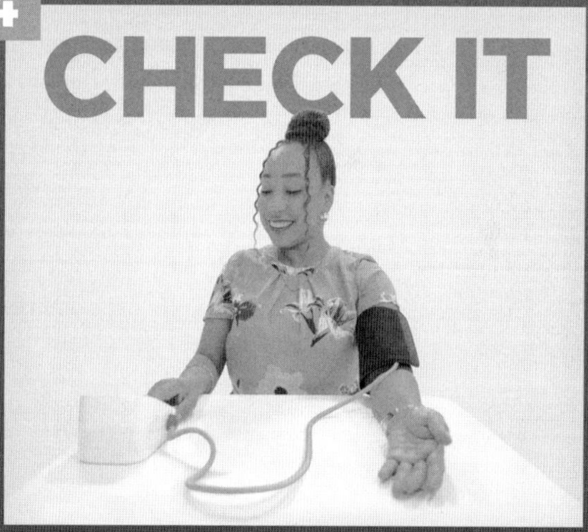

Check it every day. Self-monitoring is power.

ad COUNCIL

American Heart Association.

AMA AMERICAN MEDICAL ASSOCIATION

Visit: ManageYourBP.org

Or scan code for more.

In partnership with HHS Office of Minority Health and Health Resources and Services Administration under cooperative agreements CPIMP211227 and CPIMP211228.

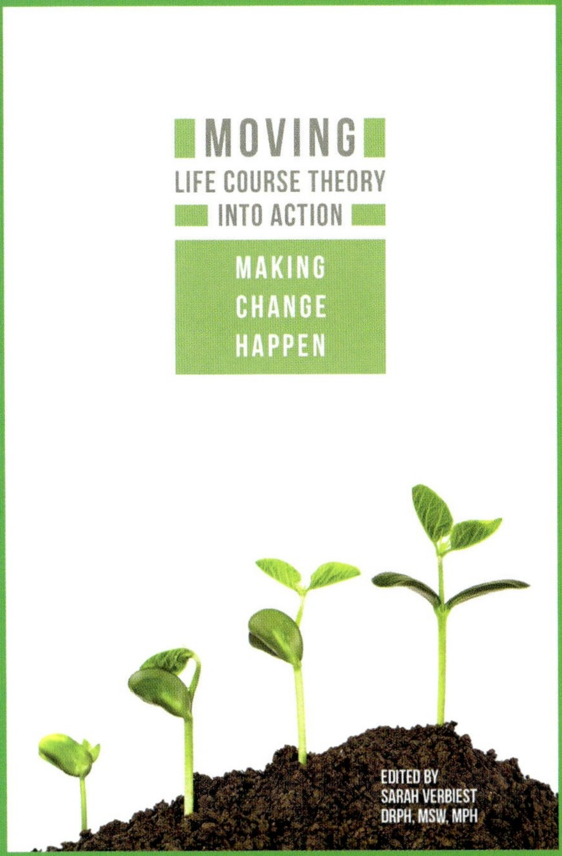

Moving Life Course Theory Into Action: *Making Change Happen*

Edited by Sarah Verbiest
DrPH, MSW, MPH

ISBN: 978-087553-2950
496 pages, Softbound, 2018

Over the past decade, practitioners in the field of maternal and child health have gained a general understanding of Life Course Theory and its potential application to practice. This book focuses on moving Life Course Theory into practice, thereby filling a need for practitioners across a variety of fields and providing them with valuable strategies on how to apply this approach.

Moving Life Course Theory Into Action is designed to fit into the busy lives of practitioners. With new ideas and strategies delivered in a compact handbook style format, each chapter includes key points that offer a quick summary of the main lessons advanced by the authors.

Order today at
aphabookstore.org

For classroom use contact
bookstoreservices@apha.org

APHA PRESS
AN IMPRINT OF **AMERICAN PUBLIC HEALTH ASSOCIATION**